Anti-Inflammatory Diet For Beginners

The Complete Beginners Guide to Heal the Immune
System, Feel Better and Restore Optimal
Health to the Cookbook not
to be missed!

I0421635

Written by Mark Sell

TABLE OF CONTENTS

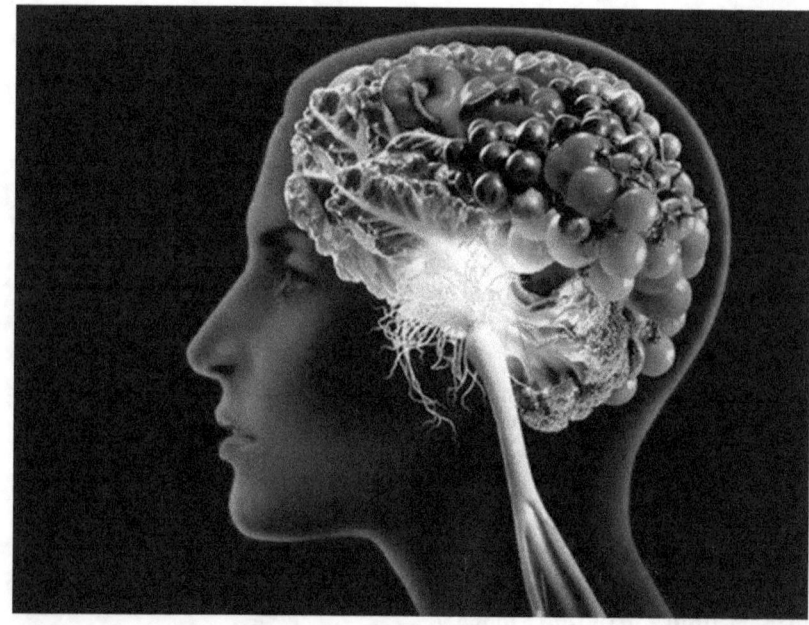

One of the most incredible and complex parts of the human body is the immune system. The immune system is able to recognize foreign substances like viruses and bacteria that might do our body harm.

It's important to know that there are two main parts of the immune system. The first is innate immunity and you are born with it totally intact; its job is to protect you against outside threats through its protective barriers like mucus and stomach acid. Fevers and the cough reflex are some other example of antigens that the innate immunity handles.

The second type of immunity makes up the adaptive immune system and it's constantly developing as you develop in life. Each time you are exposed to a germ or illness, your adaptive immune system keeps an record of it and helps your body build up a pre-programmed defense. And then, ideally, it won't make you sick the next time you come into contact with it. This adaptive immune process involves a complex system of chemicals, cells, and biological pathways that make up one of the great wonders of the human body.

The immune system and inflammation go hand in hand, and causing an inflammatory response is one major way the immune system responds to a threat and starts to fight off bacteria or tissue damage.

WHAT IS INFLAMMATION

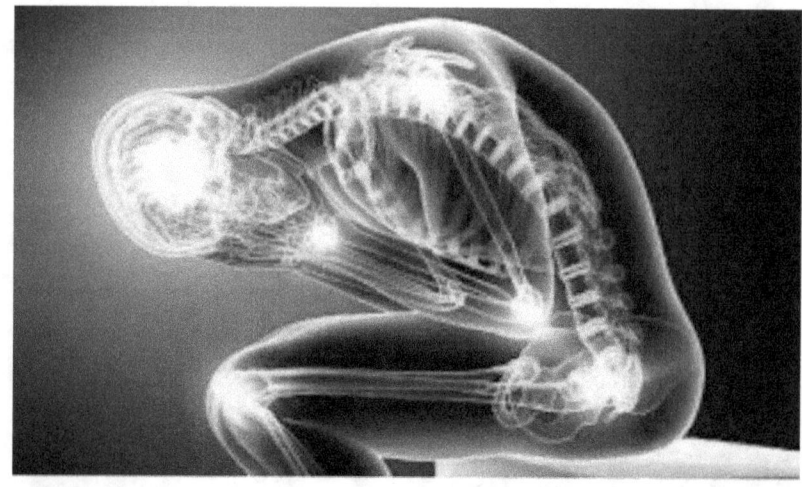

Inflammation is a natural process with the biological purpose to initiate healing by increasing circulation. It is a complex process involving both the immune system and vascular system and the interplay of various chemical mediators. Increased circulation brings white blood cells and nourishment to the site of injury or infection so that invading pathogens are killed and damage may be repaired. Characteristic signs of inflammation include pain (dolor), heat (calor), swelling (tumor) and redness (rubor).

When Inflammation Goes Awry:

While some inflammation is beneficial and appropriate for healing, chronic or excessive inflammation, serving no purpose produces damage. Chronic inflammation has a bad reputation because it is implicated in various disease processes including (but not limited to)...

- autoimmune diseases
- arthritis
- diabetes
- Alzheimer's disease
- atherosclerosis (hardening of arteries that leads to heart attack and stroke)

- ADD and ADHD
- allergies & asthma
- cancers
- inflammatory bowel disease

Soft tissue swelling and chemical mediators involved in inflammation can also irritate nerve endings, contributing to pain.

What is the Anti-Inflammatory Diet?

It is a well-known fact that different foods are metabolized differently, some promoting inflammation and others reducing it. The purpose of the anti-inflammatory diet is to promote optimal health and healing by choosing foods that reduce inflammation. If one can successfully control excessive inflammation through natural means (like through diet), it reduces one's dependence on anti-inflammatory medications that have unwanted and unhealthy side effects and don't solve the underlying problem. While anti-inflammatory medications (such as NSAIDs) is a quick fix to ease symptoms, they ultimately weaken the immune system by damaging the gastrointestinal tract which plays an important role in immune system function.

Anti-inflammatory Diet Basics:

In general, eat an abundance of fresh vegetables and fruits, whole grains, anti-inflammatory fats and nuts while limiting processed foods, meat protein, milk products, refined sugars, artificial colors/flavors/sweeteners and food sensitivities.

Vegetables:

Enjoy an abundance of fresh vegetables and fruits in a variety of colors (preferably organic). Fruits and vegetables are full of vitamins, minerals, antioxidants and fiber which give the body the essential building blocks for health. Examples include beans, squash, lintels, sweet potatoes, cruciferous vegetables, avocados, dark leafy greens... There are so many choices! As for fruits, pineapple and papaya are particularly good because they are high in bromelain, a powerful natural anti-inflammatory. Fruits and vegetables also make great, healthy snacks.

Avoid / Limit:

Avoid produce that is not grown organically. Toxic chemical residues from herbicides and pesticides can remain and when ingested are foreign irritants to the system. Many crops in

North America are also genetically engineered and are put on the market without rigorous scientific study to determine safety for human consumption. Independent research is finally being done to show toxic effects of consuming genetically modified organisms. Foreign DNA is randomly inserted into the genome of a crop. Examples include herbicide resistant corn and soy which are resistant to the herbicide Roundup, made by Monsanto. Roughly 90% of all corn and soy sold in North America is genetically modified. Also be aware of derivatives of genetically modified ingredients (such as corn starch and corn syrup etc.). It has also been suggested that consuming GMOs is a contributing factor to the rise in allergies as our bodies are recognizing these food substances as foreign. By choosing items with the "certified organic" label, you avoid both GMOs and toxic herbicides/pesticides.

For some people, vegetables in the nightshade family may pose a concern. Examples of nightshade vegetables include tomatoes, peppers, potatoes and eggplant. Nightshades contain alkaloids which are thought to exacerbate inflammation and joint damage in certain susceptible individuals with arthritis (though research is conflicting). Thus, for some individuals, limiting or avoiding nightshade vegetables may be beneficial.

Fats:

Enjoy healthy, anti-inflammatory fats including olive oil, coconut oil, avocados, nuts, salmon and sardines. In humans, there are two essential fatty acids, alpha-linolenic acid (an omega-3) and linoleic acid (an omega-6). These are "essential" because they are required for good health but the body does not synthesize them. Omega-3 fats are anti-inflammatory. Omega-6 fats can be pro-inflammatory or anti-inflammatory (as it can be metabolized by two different pathways). Researchers suggest that keeping the ratio of omega-6 to omega-3 between 2:1 and 4:1 is best for health. The modern diet tends to be high in omega-6 as it is abundantly available in cooking oils. Thus, including rich sources of omega-3 is important (such as fish, flax and walnuts especially).

Avoid / Limit:

Fats to limit or avoid include margarine, butter, shortening, hydrogenated oils, trans fats, saturated fats, and milk fat. Omega-6 fats are very high in corn oil, safflower oil and sunflower oil. Trans fats are linked with inflammatory diseases.

Meat:

In general, limit animal proteins because they tend to acidify the body and also promote inflammation. When selecting animal protein, enjoy fish, poultry (especially free-range and organically raised), lamb and omega-3 eggs.

Avoid / Limit:

Limit beef, pork, shellfish and factory farmed eggs. In general, grass-fed is superior to grain-fed. Avoid charred foods, smoked foods and cold cuts. Cold cuts contain nitrates and nitrites which promote cancer. Barbequed foods contain polycyclic aromatic hydrocarbons (PAHs) and heterocyclic amines (HCAs) which also promote cancer.

Dairy:

Enjoy dairy substitutes in moderation (such as almond milk).

Avoid / Limit:

Avoid or limit dairy products in general. This includes milk, yogurt, cheese and ice cream. As we age, we lose the enzyme that digests dairy, resulting in lactose intolerance and inflammation. The milk protein, casein, is also acidifying which (despite what many people are brought up thinking) robs the bones of calcium.

Grains:

Enjoy whole grains as opposed to refined grains. Refined grains are grains in which the germ and bran have been removed. This means there is loss of fiber, minerals and vitamins. In other words, the good stuff is removed in exchange for a longer shelf life. Some good examples of healthy grains include (organic) whole wheat/oats/bulgar/coucous, quinoa and whole oats (like steel-cut oats).

Whole grains are also a rich source of complex carbohydrates. Complex carbohydrates (as opposed to simple sugars) will prevent spikes in your blood sugar level. Sugar promotes inflammation.

Avoid / Limit:

Avoid or limit refined carbohydrates such as white bread, pastries, sweet things and pastas.

Nuts:

Enjoy nuts and nut butters such as almonds, walnuts, sesame seeds, pumpkin seeds and flax.

Avoid / Limit:

Avoid any specific nut allergies.

Beverages:

Enjoy plenty of pure, filtered water (avoiding chlorine, fluoride and other contaminants which are irritants that promote inflammation). Other great choices are lemon water and herbal teas.

Avoid / Limit:

Avoid sugary sodas, fruit juice (with sugar added) and milk.

Spices:

Many spices reduce inflammation. Some great examples are turmeric, oregano, rosemary, ginger, garlic and cinnamon. Bioflavenoids and polyphenols reduce inflammation and fight free radicals. Cayenne pepper is also anti-inflammatory, as it contains capsicum. Capsicum is often used in pain-relief creams.

Sweeteners:

Enjoy stevia, molasses, maple syrup or honey as better alternatives for refined sugar.

Avoid / Limit:

Avoid refined sugar, fructose and especially high fructose corn syrup which promote inflammation. Avoid artificial sweeteners.

Other:

Enjoy fermented foods such as kimchi, miso soup and sauerkraut. Fermented foods are probiotic and help to rebuild the immune system by supporting healthy microflora in the gut and to reduce inflammation. Fermented foods also tend to be easy to digest and are also factories for B vitamins.

Avoid / Limit:

In general, eliminate processed foods, artificial colors, artificial flavors and preservatives. Also avoid foods that you have a known sensitivity or allergy to as this promotes inflammation. Low grade sensitivities are easy to miss, so if you're unsure, have a food allergy test. Some of the most common problem foods include wheat (gluten), corn, soy, milk and nuts.

Everything we need for health, can be found in nature. We just need to choose well. If you need help and ideas of what to eat, there are plenty of anti-inflammatory diet recipe books available.

What Else Can You Do to Reduce Inflammation?

- Chiropractic care boosts immune system and reduces inflammation!
- Reduce exposure to environmental toxins (such as smoke)
- Reduce stress (5)
- Certain types of exercise reduce inflammation - specifically, long term, gradually progressive training, avoiding over-exertion (6)

ABOUT THE ANTI-INFLAMMATORY DIET

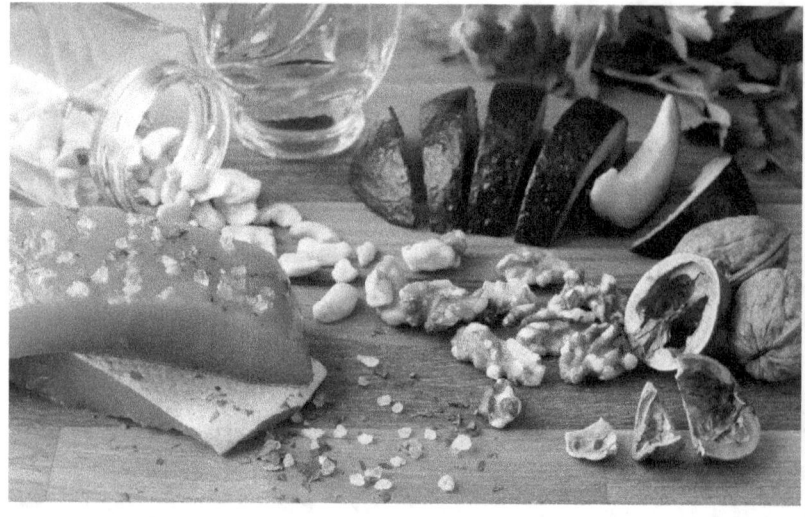

Anti-inflammatory foods are getting tons of hype these days. In fact, just about everyone is using the term "inflammation," from your cardiologist to Tom and Gisele! But keep your baloney detector on.

1 Inflammatory diets are also a thing.

The saturated fat added sugar and sodium in refined carbs and processed snacks make your body's cells work overtime to get their regular job done. Doctors can identify inflammation using biomarkers of oxidative stress, the result of biological processes that cause organ tissue damage. Diet, exercise and smoking status can affect inflammation, but so do uncontrollable causes like autoimmune diseases.

2 It's not just for weight loss.

Anti-inflammatory eating is more of a disease prevention plan. A overwhelming amount of research has shown that people who eat anti-inflammatory foods are at significantly lower risk of developing chronic disease. They're also more likely to maintain healthy weights.

3 Anti-inflammatory foods are everywhere.

The anti-inflammatory diet is often considered an Mediterranean diet, since they recommend the similar foods: Veggies, fruit, whole grains, nuts, seeds, oils, legumes, low-fat dairy and fish. The flavonoids in plants are specifically linked to protecting your body's cells from damage. Both produces and lean protein sources like beans and seafood also contain good-for-you polyunsaturated and monounsaturated fats.

4 You may have these hidden signs of inflammation.

You can't feel inflammation but, if you know what symptoms to look for, you can catch it early, before health conditions emerge. Potential inflammatory warning signs include digestive issues, intermittent joint pain, new food sensitivities, belly fat, worsening allergies, brain fog, unexplained fatigue, moodiness, sleep problems, and rashes.

5 It's inclusive, not exclusive.

Traditional diets always talk about what you can't eat, but when it comes to anti-inflammatory diets, more is more. Colorful foods like leafy greens (spinach, kale), cruciferous veggies (broccoli, cauliflower), carotenoids (tomatoes, carrots) and anthocyanins (beets, berries) are all anti-inflammatory staples.

6 You won't feel hungry.

The plant-based powerhouses known as pulses are an excellent way to incorporate antioxidant- and mineral-rich foods into your everyday life. Dry peas, beans, chickpeas and lentils combine lean protein, unsaturated fats and fiber, filling you up without messing with your diet.

7 Wine and coffee are encouraged.

When it comes to decreasing your risk of Alzheimer's, cardiovascular disease and diabetes, light to moderate alcohol intake of any kind can help. Packed with flavonoids and antioxidants, coffee beans not only ward off cognitive decline, but also boost brain function and stimulation of the central nervous system. Just steer clear of sweetened drinks sugary beverages can increase inflammation!

8 Your mood could get a boost.

Women of childbearing age eat 50% less fish than they should, largely due to previous confusion about prenatal effects. The truth is 12 ounces a week can provide a whole host of anti-inflammatory benefits. Plus, the omega-3's in fish have been linked to an lower risk of depression and reduced anxiety symptoms. Some of our favorite picks include tuna, salmon, sardines, anchovies and other white fish.

9 It's filled with flavor.

Turmeric offers powerful anti inflammatory benefits, says Dr. Corey Kirschner, of the Whole Body Cure, a anti-inflammatory diet plan from our partners at Prevention. Supercharge its anti inflammatory effects by combining it with black pepper, which helps to increase the amount of curcumin (the active ingredient in turmeric) your body can absorb. Turmeric is also fat soluble, he says, so you'll increase your absorption by combining it with a healthy fat like olive oil.

10 Cooking oils are a-okay.

Extra-virgin olive oil is filled with polyphenols, antioxidant-compounds linked to maintaining cell integrity and improving blood flow throughout your body. Canola oil, made from rapeseed, is another anti-inflammatory staple.

11 Conscious indulgences are key.

Ultimately, the anti-inflammatory diet emphasizes real foods as close to nature as possible. But since indulgence is a key part of any eating plan, try treating yourself to about 200 calories of chocolate per day. Research says that eating chocolate regularly may also help maintain a normal BMI. Plus, it can help you cut back on other processed treats.

12 You can try a whole body approach.

Prevention's Whole Body Cure includes 60+ anti-inflammatory recipes, along with the detailed advice you need to reverse chronic inflammation — no prescription required.

13 tomato salad

Just one meal or snack or heck, even a weekend full of fried food cannot induce a state of "inflammation." However, an anti-inflammatory diet may help many people lose weight because it's chock-full of nutrient-dense and delicious foods.

An Anti-Inflammatory Diet For Leaky Gut Disease

Leaky gut disease or leaky gut syndrome is a condition that can be caused by antibiotics, infections, parasites, toxins, or poor diet. The significant feature of the condition is alteration or damage to the bowel lining. As the lining becomes more permeable than normal it allows microbes, undigested food, waste, toxins, or large macromolecules to enter. Some researchers believe that these substances have a direct affect on the body; others think the problem is an immune reaction to those substances.

Whatever has caused it for you, you probably just wish the symptoms -- everything from acne and indigestion to anxiety and fatigue to joint pain and constipation, to name an few - would go away. Unfortunately, that wish can lead to treating just the symptoms. If you have Leaky Gut Disease, however, it's important that you don't just address the symptoms. You need to focus on the root causes of the condition.

One -- if not the main one -- of these root causes is diet. While practitioners disagree on an lot of things about Leaky Gut Disease (whether it even really exists, for example), the diet primarily recommended for those suffering from it - the anti-inflammatory diet - is generally acknowledged to be a healthy one for almost everyone.

The anti-inflammatory diet isn't really a diet; it's more of an eating plan. And if you do a little research, you'll find that there's not just one anti-inflammatory diet; there are several, each with a different spin. For our purposes here, I've tried to present what is a "generic" version. This version does share with the others the concept that continued and out-of-control inflammation leads to illness and that following an eating plan that avoids inflaming the body promotes health and can help prevent disease.

In general an anti-inflammatory diet includes:

Plenty of fruits and vegetables

Plenty of whole grains (e.g., brown rice, bulgur wheat)

Lean protein (e.g., chicken, fish)

Anti-inflammatory spices (e.g., curry, ginger)

Omega-3 fatty acids (such as those found in fish, fish oil supplements, and walnuts)

A reduction in

Refined carbohydrates (e,g., pasta, white rice)

Red meat and full-fat dairy foods

Saturated and trans fats

No refined or processed foods

Many who endorse this diet also urge that you avoid refined sugar and products that contain it as well as caffeine and alcohol. And while drugs don't fall into the diet category, have your doctor review your prescriptions and monitor your use of OTC drugs, especially NSAIDs.

One word of caution regarding this plan: The effects you experience (i.e., an improvement in your symptoms) will not be as immediate as they would be if you treated yourself with medications. You probably need to give the anti-inflammatory diet at least two weeks versus the hour or two an medicine might take. On the other side, this diet might have a bonus effect not usually found in medications: weight loss!

Age: Increasing age is positively correlated with elevated levels of several inflammatory molecules. The age-associated increase in inflammatory molecules may be due to mitochondrial dysfunction or free radical accumulation over time and other age-related factors like increase in visceral body fat.

Obesity: Many studies reported that fat tissue is an endocrine organ, secreting multiple adipokines and other inflammatory mediators. Some reports show that body mass index of an individual is proportional to the amount of pro-inflammatory cytokines secreted. Metabolic syndrome typifies this well.

Diet: Diet rich in saturated fat, trans-fats, or refined sugar is associated with higher production of pro-inflammatory molecules, especially in individuals with diabetes or overweight individuals.

Smoking: Cigarette smoking is associated with lowering the production of anti-inflammatory molecules and inducing inflammation.

Low Sex Hormones: Studies show that sex hormones like testosterone and estrogen can suppress the production and secretion of several pro-inflammatory markers and it has been observed that maintaining sex hormone levels reduces the risk of several inflammatory diseases.

Stress and Sleep Disorders: Both physical and emotional stress is associated with inflammatory cytokine release. Stress can also cause sleep disorders. Since individuals with irregular sleep schedules are more likely to have chronic inflammation than consistent sleepers, the sleep disorder is also considered as one of the independent risk factors for chronic inflammation.

What is chronic Inflammation?

To back up for a moment, let me give you a very brief primer on inflammation. It's a complex system in our bodies with an ever-growing list of identified components, but the big picture is that it occurs in two main ways. It can be a self-limited response to an injury or infection, for example if you get a paper-cut or a sprained ankle. You'll notice redness, pain, warmth and swelling in the area. But once all the cells from the inflammatory response have done their job and the injury is healed, that inflammation disappears. That's the kind of inflammation you want to happen.

The other kind of inflammation, called chronic inflammation, is the problematic one. It may occur if the immune system is trying to fend off an infection, like Lyme disease, but isn't having success. Or it may occur if the immune system becomes confused, such as in someone who has antibodies to gluten that also end up attacking other parts of the body that resemble gluten. Inflammation also happens when the immune system senses that something isn't right, such as when LDL cholesterol makes its way into the lining of an artery. White blood cells follow, but instead of fixing the problem, they inadvertently make it worse by making the plaque unstable and more likely to rupture

Symptoms of Chronic Inflammation

Some of the common signs and symptoms that develop during chronic inflammation are listed below.

Body pain

Constant fatigue and insomnia

Depression, anxiety and mood disorders

Gastrointestinal complications like constipation, diarrhea, and acid reflux

Weight gain

Frequent infections

Evaluation

Tests for Chronic Inflammation

Unfortunately, there are no highly effective laboratory measures to assess patients for chronic inflammation and diagnoses are only undertaken when the inflammation occurs in association with another medical condition.

The best test to confirm clinically chronic inflammation is serum protein electrophoresis (SPE) which shows concomitant hypoalbuminemia and polyclonal increase in all gamma globulins (polyclonal gammopathy).

The two blood tests that are inexpensive and good markers of systemic inflammation include high-sensitivity C-reactive protein (hsCRP) and fibrinogen. High levels of hs-CRP indicate inflammation, but it is not a specific marker for chronic inflammation since it is also elevated in acute inflammation resulting from a recent injury or sickness. The normal serum levels for hsCRP is less than 0.55 mg/L in men and less than 1.0 mg/L in women. The normal levels of fibrinogen are 200 to 300 mg/dl. SAA (Serum Amyloid A) can also mark inflammation but is not a standardized test.

Detecting pro-inflammatory cytokines like tumor necrosis factor-alpha (TNF-alpha), interleukin-1 beta (IL-1beta), interleukin-6 (IL-6), and interleukin-8 (IL-8) is an expensive method but may identify specific factors causing chronic inflammation. Again, the assays are not standardized like hs-CRP, fibrinogen, and SPE.

Treatment / Management

Many dietary and lifestyle changes may be helpful in removing inflammation triggers and reducing chronic inflammation as listed below. The most effective is weight loss.

Low-glycemic diet: Diet with a high glycemic index is related to high risk of stroke, coronary heart disease, and type 2 diabetes mellitus. It is beneficial to limit consumption of inflammation-promoting foods like sodas, refined carbohydrates, fructose corn syrup in a diet.

Reduce intake of total, saturated fat and trans fats: Some dietary saturated and synthetic trans-fats aggravate inflammation, while omega-3 polyunsaturated fats appear to be anti-inflammatory. Processed and packaged foods that contain trans fats such as processed seed and vegetable oils, baked goods (like soybean and corn oil) should be reduced from the diet.

Fruits and vegetables: Blueberries, apples, Brussels sprouts, cabbage, broccoli, and cauliflower, that are high in natural antioxidants and polyphenols and other anti-inflammatory compounds, may protect against inflammation.

Fiber: High intake of dietary soluble and insoluble fiber is associated with lowering levels of IL-6 and TNF-alpha.

Nuts: such as almonds is associated with lowering risk of cardiovascular disease and diabetes.

Green and black tea polyphenols: Tea polyphenols are associated with a reduction in CRP in human clinical studies.

Curcumin: a constituent of turmeric causes significant patient improvements in several inflammatory diseases especially in animal models.

Fish Oil: The richest source of the omega-3 fatty acids. Higher intake of omega-3 fatty acids is associated with lowering levels of TNF-alpha, CRP, and IL-6.

Mung bean: Rich in flavonoids (particularly vitexin and isovitexin). It is traditional food and herbal medicine known for its anti-inflammatory effects.

Micronutrients: Magnesium, vitamin D, vitamin E, zinc and selenium). Magnesium is listed as one of the most anti-inflammatory dietary factors, and its intake is associated with lowering of hsCRP, IL-6, and TNF-alpha activity. Vitamin D exerts its anti-inflammatory activity by suppressing inflammatory mediators such as prostaglandins and nuclear factor kappa-light-chain-enhancer of activated B cells. Vitamin E, zinc, and selenium act as antioxidants in the body.

Sesame Lignans: Sesame oil consumption reduces the synthesis of prostaglandin, leukotrienes, and thromboxanes and is known for its potential hypotensive activity.

Physical Exercise

In human clinical trials, it is shown that energy expenditure through exercise lowers multiple pro-inflammatory molecules and cytokines independently of weight loss.

Conventional Drugs to Combat Chronic Inflammation

Metformin is commonly used in the treatment of type II diabetic patients with dyslipidemia and low-grade inflammation. The anti-inflammatory activity of Metformin is evident by reductions in circulating TNF-alpha, IL-1beta, CRP, and fibrinogen in these patients.

Non-steroidal anti-inflammatory drugs (NSAIDs) like naproxen, ibuprofen, and aspirin acts by inhibiting an enzyme cyclooxygenase (COX) that contributes to inflammation and are mostly used to alleviate the pain caused by inflammation in patients with arthritis.

Statins are anti-inflammatory as they reduce multiple circulating and cellular biomediators of inflammation. This pleiotropic effect appears to contribute in part to the reduction in cardiovascular events.

Corticosteroids also prevent several mechanisms involved in inflammation. Glucocorticoids are prescribed for inflammatory conditions including inflammatory arthritis, systemic lupus, sarcoidosis, and asthma.

Herbal supplements like ginger, turmeric, cannabis, hyssop, and Harpagophytum procumbens are shown to have anti-inflammatory properties however one should always consult with a doctor before their use and caution should be taken for using some herbs like hyssop and cannabis.

Differential Diagnosis

It is important to realize that chronic inflammation is not a specific disease but a mechanistic process. The diseases associated with chronic inflammation are multiple and include CVD, diabetes, malignancy, auto-immune disease, chronic hepatic and renal disease, etc. Hence a good history, physical examination, and routine laboratory tests (glucose, creatinine, liver function, rheumatoid factor, complete blood count, antinuclear antibodies) can confirm or rule out most of the differential diagnoses. Also, pertinent imaging studies will be helpful in certain circumstances, e.g., Inflammatory bowel disease or serum protein electrophoresis for polyclonal gammopathy.

Complications

Although chronic inflammation progresses silently, it is the cause of most chronic diseases and presents a major threat to the health and longevity of individuals. Inflammation is considered a major contributor to several diseases.

Cardiovascular diseases: Many clinical studies have shown strong and consistent relationships between markers of inflammation such as hsCRP and cardiovascular disease prediction. Furthermore, Atherosclerosis is a pro-inflammatory state with all the features of chronic low-grade inflammation and leads to increase cardiovascular events such as myocardial infarction, stroke, among others.

Cancer: Chronic low-level inflammation also appears to participate in many types of cancer such as kidney, prostate, ovarian, hepatocellular, pancreatic, colorectal, lung, and mesothelioma.

Diabetes: Immune cells like macrophages infiltrate pancreatic tissues releasing pro-inflammatory molecules in diabetic individuals. Both are circulating and cellular biomarkers underscore that diabetes is a chronic inflammatory disease. Chronic complications linked with diabetes include both microvascular and macrovascular complications. Diabetes not only increases the risk of macrovascular complications like strokes and heart attacks but also the microvascular complications like diabetic retinopathy, neuropathy, and nephropathy.

Rheumatoid arthritis: It is thought to be initiated by an infectious agent or an environmental factor like exposure to cigarette smoke which induces a local inflammatory response in joints, infiltration of immune cells and release of cytokines.

Allergic asthma: A complex, chronic inflammatory disorder associated with inappropriate immune response and inflammation in conducting airways involving a decline in airway function and tissue remodeling.

Chronic obstructive pulmonary disease (COPD): An obstructive lung disease, develops as a chronic inflammatory response to inspired irritants and characterized by long-term breathing problems.

Alzheimer: In older adults, chronic low-level inflammation is linked to cognitive decline and dementia.

Chronic kidney disease (CKD): Low-grade inflammation is a common feature of chronic kidney disease. It can lead to the retention of several pro-inflammatory molecules in the blood and contributes to the progression of CKD and mortality.

Inflammatory Bowel Disease (IBD) is a group of chronic inflammatory disorders of the digestive tract. It can develop as ulcerative colitis causing long-lasting inflammation and ulcers in the lining of large intestine and rectum or Crohn's disease characterized by inflammation of the lining of digestive tract dispersing into affected tissues such as mouth, esophagus, stomach and the anus.

Deterrence and Patient Education

Chronic inflammation can have a deleterious effect on the body and is a key factor causing almost all chronic degenerative diseases. The following are some of the most effective ways to prevent chronic inflammation.

Increase uptake of anti-inflammatory foods: It is important to avoid eating simple sugars, refined carbohydrates, high-glycemic foods, trans fats, and hydrogenated oils. Consuming whole grains, natural foods, plenty of vegetables and fruits such as avocados, cherries, kale, and fatty fish like salmon is helpful in defeating inflammation.

Minimize intake of antibiotics and NSAIDs: Use of antibiotics, antacids, and NSAIDs should be avoided as it could harm the microbiome in the gut causing inflammation in intestinal walls known as leaky gut which in turn releases toxins and triggers chronic, body-wide inflammation.

Exercise regularly to maintain an optimum weight: It is largely known that adipose tissue in obese or overweight individuals induces low-grade systemic inflammation. Regular exercise is helpful not only in controlling weight but also decreasing the risk of cardiovascular diseases and strengthening the heart, muscles, and bones.

Sleep longer: Overnight sleep (ideally at least 7 to 8 hours) helps stimulating human growth hormones and testosterone in the body to rebuild itself.

Stress Less: Chronic psychological stress is linked to greater risk for depression, heart disease and body losing its ability to regulate the inflammatory response and normal defense. Yoga and meditation are helpful in alleviating stress-induced inflammation and its harmful effects on the body.

Features

Most of the features of acute inflammation continue as the inflammation becomes chronic, including expansion of blood vessels (vasodilation), increase in blood flow, capillary permeability and migration of neutrophils into the infected tissue through the capillary wall (diapedesis). However, the composition of the white blood cells changes soon and the macrophages and lymphocytes begin to replace short-lived neutrophils. Thus the hallmarks of chronic inflammation are the infiltration of the primary inflammatory cells such as macrophages, lymphocytes, and plasma cells in the tissue site, producing inflammatory cytokines, growth factors, enzymes and hence contributing to the progression of tissue damage and secondary repair including fibrosis and granuloma formation, etc.

Types of Chronic Inflammation

Nonspecific proliferative: Characterized by the presence of non-specific granulation tissue formed by infiltration of mononuclear cells (lymphocytes, macrophages, plasma cells) and proliferation of fibroblasts, connective tissue, vessels and epithelial cells, for example, an inflammatory polyp-like nasal or cervical polyp and lung abscess.

Granulomatous inflammation: A specific type of chronic inflammation characterized by the presence of distinct nodular lesions or granulomas formed with an aggregation of activated macrophages or its derived cell called epithelioid cells usually surrounded by lymphocytes. The macrophages or epithelioid cells inside the granulomas often coalesce to form Langhans or giant cells such as foreign body, Aschoff, Reed-Sternberg and Tumor giant cells. There are two types:

Granuloma formed due to a foreign body or T-cell mediated immune response is termed as foreign body granuloma, for example, silicosis

Granuloma that are formed from chronic infection is termed as infectious granuloma, for example, tuberculosis and leprosy.

5 SIGNS TO LOOK OUT FOR

If you are striving to keep yourself healthy for now and many years to come, and you want to know what single thing you should be paying attention to more than anything else, it is this: inflammation.

The reason inflammation is so critical is that it has been found to be a player in almost every chronic disease. And if it hasn't been shown to be associated with a chronic disease, it's probably just because no one has looked for it.

You probably wouldn't be surprised to hear that it is an major part of autoimmune diseases since they are all directly caused by the immune system. Maybe you've also already heard that the white cells that sneak into the walls of your arteries are major contributors to cardiovascular disease, meaning it's not just about cholesterol build-up. Perhaps you also know that cancer tends to form in areas that are chronically inflamed. But you might not have expected inflammation to be a component of osteoarthritis, the disease that we doctors thought was just from too much tackle football or tennis (wear and tear of the bones). Inflammation even plays an role in hypertension and depression.

Top 5 Symptoms of Chronic Inflammation

At Parsley Health, one of our main goals is to help people prevent and reverse chronic disease, so we pay an lot of attention to chronic inflammation. We look for symptoms of inflammation beginning at our patients' very first visit. Here are five common indications that someone may have a chronic inflammatory condition:

Body pain, especially in the joints

Skin rashes, such as eczema or psoriasis

Excessive mucus production (ie, always needing to clear your throat or blow your nose)

Low energy, despite sufficient sleep

Poor digestion, including bloating, abdominal pain, constipation and loose stool

We're diving deep into inflammation. Get our newsletter to read every piece as it's published.

The Tests Your Doctor Should Be Doing

Not only do we listen for inflammation in our patients' histories, but we also test for it in every patient we see using these three biomarkers:

White blood cell count

Sedimentation rate (ESR)

High sensitivity c-reactive protein (hsCRP). (Note: About 1/3 of the adult U.S. population has an elevated CRP.)

Each one of these looks at different components of the blood to see if there is inflammation in the body. They are non-specific, meaning they don't tell us where the inflammation is coming from, but they do clue us in to look harder for it. Taken together, we get a pretty good idea as to whether inflammation is an issue, and we can also use them to track if the inflammation is resolving or worsening.

How to Heal Chronic Inflammation

If all this talk of chronic inflammation and its pervasive effect on chronic disease is getting you nervous, don't worry! You actually don't need to know which cytokine blocks which receptor to know what to do.

Our recommended approach is very similar to what we recommend for health in general:

Remove the foods that are known to cause inflammation, like sugar, dairy and simple carbohydrates.

Avoid foods that you are sensitive to. This is something we often test for or figure out with an elimination diet.

Eat lots of foods that are known to be anti-inflammatory, like leafy greens, colorful veggies, nuts, seeds, herbs and spices (eg, turmeric, ginger and rosemary) and extra virgin olive oil.

Exercise. Regular exercise of moderate intensity improves immune function and decreases inflammation.(Even occasional exercise has benefits, but high-intensity exercise may actually have a detrimental effect on the immune system.)

Minimize stress and optimize how you respond to it.

Supplements such as probiotics, turmeric, resveratrol and fish oil are known to help fight inflammation.

Inflammation is an amazing unifier of most chronic diseases, so if you want to optimize your current and future health, you can do so by minimizing inflammation. Take note if you have symptoms that seem consistent with inflammation, check for it with blood tests, and do your best to adopt an anti-inflammatory lifestyle.

Ways To Reduce Inflammation

I started connecting the dots between my diet and lifestyle, chronic inflammation, and disease, an light bulb turned on. Why? Because our daily choices are at the root of chronic inflammation.

Over the past decade, I've renovated everything from my grocery cart to my makeup bag to my mind in an effort to upgrade my immune system. And as I moved from a stressful life full of fast food, toxins, and bad boyfriends to an more balanced existence filled with plant-passionate nourishment, inner growth, and conscious living, I started experiencing the perks. Chronic inflammation decreased and my body started working with me to heal and rebuild.

Want to start connecting the dots in your own life? First, let's learn about acute and chronic inflammation, since they play very different roles in our everyday health. Then, we'll cover the causes of chronic inflammation and how to reduce its impact on your health.

The Results of Chronic Inflammation

Over time, chronic inflammation wears out your immune system, leading to chronic diseases and other health issues including cancer, asthma, autoimmune diseases, allergies, irritable bowel syndrome, arthritis, osteoporosis, and even (gasp!) appearing older than your years.

Unfortunately, these challenges are often only treated with drugs and surgery, which may provide temporary relief from the symptoms, but do not treat the root of the problem. In addition, these drugs and their side effects sometimes only add to your health problems.

Could it be that many of the pills in your cabinet are just Band-Aids and that the key to health lies in your daily diet and lifestyle choices? That's certainly what I've found to be true.

The integrative MDs I know and trust are helping their patients identify and address their health issues by looking at the way they lead their lives and nipping their inflammation-happy habits in the bud. If possible, find an integrative doctor who can help you along the way and target your unique needs. They can also test your blood for inflammation make sure your doc requests a CRP—C-reactive Protein test.

Although this may seem overwhelming, it's actually the opposite. The following tips will empower you and help you reduce inflammation over time. Try an few (or just one) of these suggestions on for size and see how you feel. As always, slow and steady wins the race, or in this case, puts out the fire.

How to Reduce Chronic Inflammation

1. Eat more plant-based, whole, nutrient-dense foods.

Crowd out the inflammatory foods we discussed above (refined sugar and flour, processed junk, animal products, etc.) by adding a variety of plant-based whole foods to your diet. These foods will flood your body with the vitamins, minerals, cancer-fighting phytochemicals, antioxidants, and fiber it needs to recover from chronic inflammation.

2. Focus on gut health.

Your gut holds approximately 60 to 70 percent of your immune system, so it stands to reason that it would be a great place to reduce chronic inflammation. And if your gut is in bad shape, you can only imagine that your immune system is in some serious trouble. Check out my tips for improving gut health here. A great way to start is by taking a daily probiotic.

3. Identify and address food allergies and chronic (or hidden) infections.

You could be fighting an losing battle if you're ignoring potential food sensitivities and/or infections. If your body is working to cope and fight these challenges every day, you can bet that you're stoking the fires of inflammation on a regular basis.

Gluten, soy, dairy, eggs, and yeast are common food allergens that might be distracting your immune system every time you sit down for an meal. These allergies can be identified with a blood test. Ask your doctor about testing for food allergies.

Become a symptoms detective. Only you can determine how you feel when you eat, which is where a elimination diet comes in handy. While following the elimination approach, you remove all common allergens from your diet and then slowly reintroduce them, one by one. Talk to your doc about these options, and do some independent research at Google University.

Another possibility worth exploring is chronic infection (bacteria, viruses, yeast, parasites). These guys could be hiding out in your body just under the radar and dragging your immune system down. You have a couple options for testing—look at your bloodwork and/or your poop. It may not be pretty, but knowledge is power, so be brave and have your stool checked. You can have your stool analyzed—this analysis will identify parasites, abnormal bacteria, yeasts, and other gastrointestinal issues, which will help you create a game plan that targets the infection, ideally with the help of an integrative MD or naturopath.

You may also want to look into Leaky Gut Syndrome, a condition that can result in damage to your intestinal lining. When this occurs, bacteria, undigested food, and other toxins can literally leak into your bloodstream, triggering an autoimmune response and a host of painful inflammatory symptoms. A simple urine test can tell you if you need to plug up those leaks, so to speak.

4. Relax and rest more.

Your body is hard at work repairing and restoring your glorious cells while you sleep. Most doctors recommend 7 to 8 hours of sleep per night. If you're cutting corners in the snooze department, you're cheating your immune system, which means it needs to kick into high gear in an effort to keep you well (hello, inflammation).

Stress goes hand in hand with an lack of sleep and a laundry list of demands from daily life. Unfortunately, when you're stressed out all the time, you're also producing more of the hormone cortisol inflammation's BFF. It stands to reason that you can easily reduce chronic inflammation by focusing on stress reduction, whether it's through more sleep, yoga, meditation, long walks, less technology, or a much-needed vacation. You know I love to take every opportunity I can to remind you to take a chill pill.

5. Reduce toxins in your food, home, and personal care products.

Your body's alarm system goes off when you absorb toxic chemicals and pesticides through your digestive tract and your skin. Cut down your exposure by eating organic foods whenever possible and choosing non-toxic personal care and cleaning products.

THE FUNGUS ANTI-INFLAMMATORY DIET AND HOW IT MAY TREAT YOUR NAIL FUNGUS

What is nail fungus?

The anti-inflammatory diet can help boost your immune system, which can help fight off fungal infections. Drinking the recommended six to eight glasses of water a day is suggested with this diet, which can help to cleanse your inner system, also helping to fight off infection.

In addition to being helpful in the fight to rid oneself of a fungus infection, there are other health benefits attached to the diet such as help with depression and improved mental state, a stronger immune system, less water retainage and more.

What is the Anti-Inflammatory Diet?

The anti-inflammatory diet usually consists of eating 2,000 to 3,000 calories a day. The amount of calories depends on your size. You should be eating 40 to 50% of carbohydrates, 30 % of fat and include carbohydrates, fat and protein with each meal.

This diet uses an lot of fish and fresh fruits and vegetables while minimizing the consumption of fast food meals.   Beans, winter squashes and sweet potatoes are also a big part of this diet.

This diet is not typically meant for weight loss, but can be used for health reasons and is said to help with fungal problems.

How do I know if it's working?

It may take an little while for the diet to work. Remember, if you've been eating a totally different diet, particularly if it was a poor diet, it will take a while for your system to be completely cleaned out. You might want to make a visit to a nutritionist or the local health food store to discuss how and when the diet will work.

You can expect any treatment to take six to twelve weeks to work and the change in your diet alone may not be enough. Keep a journal of what you eat and do and any changes you see if you are unsure of the effectiveness of treatment.

Okay, I'm on the diet, what else should I be doing?

Again, this is something to be discussed with your healthcare physician, a dietitian or nutritionist or even your health foot store representative who is well-versed in dietary needs. At times, a health foot store may have different or more reliable information than the internet or even your physician's office and may be able to give you some supplements, topical creams or organic lacquers which may prove to be extremely effective, especially in conjunction with the anti-inflammatory diet.

You may also want to check your library or local book store. Internet research can be helpful when making a decision regarding informational books on nail fungus and diet-related and other organic treatment remedies.

THE EASIEST CHANGES TO BOOST HEALTH

There are an million and one trendy diets out there offering to change how you look and feel in an matter of days. The consumer is flooded with products that will make their skin "appear" healthier and softer to touch. In a world with too much focus on looking good and "appearing" healthier, there is one diet that WILL make you healthier and potentially live an longer life in your anti-aged body.

The anti-inflammatory diet has so many uses today it is surprising every one of the health, fitness and beauty gurus have not jumped on the simplest of diet changes and marketed them as the next big trend in weight loss, beauty and anti-aging. The fact is the anti-inflammatory diet can do everything other diets claim they can do and increase lifespan in the process.

So how do I jump start the anti-inflammatory diet?

Think of this first week as a natural eating time, so don't make any changes or eat anything you would not normally eat. Once the list is complete, head off to the Internet for an little research and education on the power of food over inflammation. Many people are surprised by the effects seemingly healthy foods can have on overall body health and the prevention of illness. Sure, the market screams at the consumer about drinking more vitamin C and reducing calories, but what about the foods that seem healthy but really aren't? These foods will be found after a week of journaling before starting your anti-inflammatory diet.

Are there any baked foods on the list? Chances are, if these foods were purchased prepackaged; they will contain at least a small amount of trans fats. Even the small, 100 calorie bites of cupcake marketed as healthy alternatives can contain up to 0.5 grams of trans fats. Eating just two of these little cakes a day for a week contributes a whopping 7 grams of trans fats - the only healthy level is 0 grams.

Did you eat a salad this week? Many people think eating a salad is a healthy alternative and it can be, without that fat laden dressing covering the healthy greens. One tablespoon of regular dressing can contain 100 calories and about 10 grams of fat. The typical true serving is about ¼ cup per salad. That equates to 400 calories, 40 grams of fat and a -76 rating on the inflammation factor scale which measures the total inflammatory effect of foods on the body.

EATING ANTI-INFLAMMATORY FOODS

Are there really diets out there that can reduce inflammation? Do they work? Scientists have found that there is a relationship, in part, between what we eat and inflammation. They've even identified some compounds in food that can reduce inflammation and others that promote it. There is still an lot to learn about just how diet and inflammation interact, and research, as of yet, is not at that point where a specific foods or groups of foods can be singled out as being beneficial for people with arthritis. We are beginning to get a clearer picture of how eating the right way can reduce inflammation.

So why are we so concerned about inflammation? Inflammation is the body's natural defense to infections and injuries. When something goes wrong the body's immune system goes to work to inflame the area, which serves to get rid of the invader or to heal the wound. Inflammation can cause pain, swelling, redness, and warmth, but this goes away as soon as the problem is solved. This is good inflammation.

Then we have chronic inflammation, the type that's familiar to people with rheumatoid arthritis (RA), lupus, psoriatic arthritis, and other types of "inflammatory" arthritis. Chronic inflammation is the type that will not go away. All the types of arthritis that are mentioned above are a disorder of the immune system creates inflammation and then doesn't know when to shut off. Inflammatory arthritis, chronic inflammation can have serious consequences, permanent disability and tissue damage can be one if it isn't treated properly. Inflammation has been linked to a full host of other medical conditions.

Inflammation has been found to contribute to atherosclerosis, which is when fat builds up on the lining of arteries, raising the risk of heart attacks. Also, high levels of inflammation proteins have been found in the blood of people with heart disease. Inflammation has also been linked to obesity, diabetes, asthma, depression, and even Alzheimer disease and cancer. Scientists thinks that a constant level of inflammation in the body, even if the level is low, can have a number of negative effects. Research shows that diet can reduce inflammation; in theory an inflammation-lowering diet should have an effect on a wide range of health conditions.

Researchers have looked for clues in the eating habits of our early ancestors to discover which foods might benefit us the most. They believe those habits are more in tune to our eating habits with how the body processes and uses what we eat and drink. Our ancestor's diet consisted of wild lean meats (venison or boar) and wild plants (green leafy vegetables, fruits, nuts, and berries). There were no cereal grains until the agriculture revolution (about 10,000 years ago). There was very little dairy, and there were no processed or refined foods. Our diets are usually are high in meat, saturated (or bad) fats, and processed foods, and there is very little exercise. Nearly everything we eat is available close by or was as far away as our computer and the click of a mouse.

Our diet and lifestyles are way out of whack with how our bodies are made from the inside out. While our genetic make-up has changed very little from our early beginnings, our diet and lifestyles have changed a great deal and the changes have gotten worse over the last 50 to 100 years. Our genes haven't had a chance to adapt. We aren't giving our bodies the right kind of fuel, it's as though we think of our bodies as engines in a jet plane when instead they are like the engine in the very first planes. There are some foods that we are putting into our bodies, especially because we are eating way too much of them, that are affecting our health in a bad way.

There are two nutrients in our diets that have attracted attention, are omega-3 fatty acids and omega-6 fatty acids have been part of our diets for thousands of years. They are components in just about all of our many cells and are important for normal growth and development. Both of these acids play an role in inflammation. In several studies it was found that certain sources of omega 3's in particular, help to reduce the inflammation process and that omega 6's will raise it.

Now this is the problem, the average American eats on average about 15 times more omega 6's than omega 3's. While our very early ancestor's ate omega 6's and omega 3's in equal ratio, and it is believed that this is what helped to balance their ability to turn inflammation on and off. The imbalance of omega 3's and omega 6's in our diets is believed to contribute to the excess of inflammation in our bodies.

So why is it that we eat so many omega 6's now? Vegetable oils such as corn oil, safflower oil, sunflower oil, cottonseed oil, soybean oil, and the products made from them, such as margarine, are loaded with omega 6's. Even many of the processed snack foods that are so readily available today are full of these oils. Based on the best information of the time, was to use vegetable oils like those mentioned above instead of foods with saturated fats such as butter and lard. It looks like the consequences of that advice may have contributed to the increased consumption of omega 6's and therefore causing a imbalance of omega 3's and omega 6's.

You can find omega 6's in other common foods such as meats and egg yolks. The omega 6 found in meat is the fatty acids that come from grain-fed animals such as cows, lambs, pigs and chickens. Most of the meat sold in America is grain fed unlike their grass-fed cousins who contain less of those fatty acids. Wild game such as venison and boar are lower in omega 6's and fat and higher in omega 3's than the meat that comes from the supermarkets where we shop.

You can get omega 3s in both animal and plant food. Our bodies can convert omega 3s from animal sources into anti-inflammatory compounds more easily than the omega 3s from plant sources. Plant foods contain hundreds of other healthful compounds many of which that are anti-inflammatory, so don't discount them all together.

There are many foods that are high in omega 3s and that include fatty fish, especially fish from cold waters. Of course everyone knows about salmon but did you know that you can also find omega 3s in mackerel, anchovies, sardines, herring, striped bass, and bluefish. It's also widely known that wild fish are better sources of omega 3s than the farm raised ones. You can also buy eggs that have been enriched with omega 3 oils. There are several excellent sources of omega 3s in plants that are leafy greens (like kale, Swiss chard, and spinach) as well as flaxseed, wheat germ, walnuts, and their oils.

You can also get omega 3s in supplements (often as fish oil); this source has been shown to be beneficial in some instances. You should take with your doctor before you take an fish oil supplement because it can interact with some medications and under certain circumstances can increase the risk of bleeding. I take a prescribed omega 3 supplement because my doctor had told me that the ones you get in the supermarket or health food store are not pure, they have other additives that do absolutely nothing to help. There are other fats that are contributors to clogged arteries, the "bad" or saturated fats found in meats and high-fat dairy foods, these are called pro-inflammatory.

There are also the Trans fats that are relatively new to the cause of heart disease. These Trans fats can be found in processed convenience and snack foods and can be spotted by reading the labels. They can be identified as partially hydrogenated oils, often soybean oil or cottonseed oil. But, they can also occur naturally in small amounts in animal foods. The thought is that they contribute to the pro-inflammatory activities in our bodies and the amounts we eat today are staggering.

Antioxidants are substances that prevent inflammation causing "free radicals" from over taking our bodies. Plant foods such as fruits, vegetables (including beans), nuts, and seeds carry high amounts of antioxidants. Extra-virgin olive oil and walnut oil are very good sources of antioxidants, also. These foods have long been considered the basics for good health, and can be found in fruits and vegetables with colorful and vibrant pigments. The more colorful the plant, the better they are for you, from green vegetables, especially leafy ones, to low-starch vegetables, such as broccoli and cauliflower, to berries, tomatoes, and brightly colored orange and yellow fruits and vegetables.

I bet you're wondering what this has to do with Arthritis. Well, there has been some research on diet and arthritis, mostly focusing on RA. There was a study that looked into a bunch of other studies on diet and RA and found that diets high in omega 3's had some effect on reducing the symptoms of RA. There was yet another study published in 2008, that found eating omega 6 fatty acids and omega 3 fatty acids in an ratio of 2 or 3 to 1 (a low ratio compared to the 15 to 1 ratio in most people's diet) decreased the inflammation in people with RA. There was also another study that found taking omega 3 may also allow people to reduce their use of no steroidal anti-inflammatory drugs (NSAIDs), such as ibuprofen (Advil, Motrin) and naproxen (Aleve). But these and other studies don't offer enough evidence to prove that there is any particular anti-inflammatory diet that can have an real impact on arthritis symptoms. It doesn't mean that the diets are harmful; it just means that there may come a day when research may be able to prove their benefits. In the future, diet may be considered one of the many tools along with exercise and medicine that can be used to ease the symptoms of arthritis.

We don't have to revert back completely to the caveman to eat the anti-inflammatory way to benefit from the anti-inflammatory diet. Just eating a healthful diet that is recommended today is right on track. Our chief strategy should be to balance the amount of modern day foods with the foods of long ago, which were rich in the inflammation reducing foods. Really, all we have to do is replace foods rich in omega 6 with foods rich in omega 3, cutting down on how much meat and poultry we eat while eating oily fish a couple of times a week and adding more varieties of colorful fruits and vegetables, and while whole grains were not a part of our early ancestor's diet, it should be included in ours. Be sure that it is whole grains and not refined grains because they contain many beneficial nutrients and inflammation-tempering compounds. Researchers have found that eating an lot of foods high in sugar and white flour may promote inflammation, although there is more studying that needs to be done on the subject.

The amounts of knowledge we have on how the body works and how our ancestor's ate is helping to confirm the old adage: "You are what you eat." But, there is still more we need to learn before we can prescribe any one anti-inflammatory diet. Our genetic makeup and the severity of our health condition will determine the benefits we get from an anti-inflammatory diet and unfortunately there is doubt that there will be one diet that fits us all.

Also, what we eat or don't eat is just a small part of the whole story. We are not as physically active as our ancestors and physical activity has its own anti-inflammatory effects. Our ancestors were also much leaner than we are and body fat is active tissue that can make inflammatory producing compounds.

Anti-inflammatory eating is a way of selecting foods that are more in tune with what the body actually needs. We can achieve an more balanced diet by going back to our roots. If you look at the diet of the people of the Bible, you will find that they, like our caveman ancestors, were more active and their diets consisted of much the same things as our caveman ancestors. They also had no choice but to walk everywhere they wanted to go, there was no such thing as cars or trucks. While we have it easier today, our health has suffered greatly from it.

FOODS THAT FIGHT INFLAMMATION

Your immune system becomes activated when your body recognizes anything that is foreign such as an invading microbe, plant pollen, or chemical. This often triggers a process called inflammation. Intermittent bouts of inflammation directed at truly threatening invaders protect your health.

However, sometimes inflammation persists, day in and day out, even when you are not threatened by a foreign invader. That's when inflammation can become your enemy. Many major diseases that plague us including cancer, heart disease, diabetes, arthritis, depression, and Alzheimer's have been linked to chronic inflammation.

Choose the right anti-inflammatory foods, and you may be able to reduce your risk of illness. Consistently pick the wrong ones, and you could accelerate the inflammatory disease process.

Foods that cause inflammation

Try to avoid or limit these foods as much as possible:

refined carbohydrates, such as white bread and pastries

French fries and other fried foods

soda and other sugar-sweetened beverages

red meat (burgers, steaks) and processed meat (hot dogs, sausage)

margarine, shortening, and lard.

The health risks of inflammatory foods

Not surprisingly, the same foods on an inflammation diet are generally considered bad for our health, including sodas and refined carbohydrates, as well as red meat and processed meats.

"Some of the foods that have been associated with an increased risk for chronic diseases such as type 2 diabetes and heart disease are also associated with excess inflammation. "It's not surprising, since inflammation is a important underlying mechanism for the development of these diseases."

Unhealthy foods also contribute to weight gain, which is itself a risk factor for inflammation. Yet in several studies, even after researchers took obesity into account, the link between foods and inflammation remained, which suggests weight gain isn't the sole driver. "Some of the food components or ingredients may have independent effects on inflammation over and above increased caloric intake,

Anti-inflammatory foods

A anti-inflammatory diet should include these foods:

tomatoes

olive oil

green leafy vegetables, such as spinach, kale, and collards

nuts like almonds and walnuts

fatty fish like salmon, mackerel, tuna, and sardines

fruits such as strawberries, blueberries, cherries, and oranges

Benefits of anti-inflammatory foods

On the flip side are beverages and foods that reduce inflammation, and with it, chronic disease, He notes in particular fruits and vegetables such as blueberries, apples, and leafy greens that are high in natural antioxidants and polyphenols—protective compounds found in plants.

Studies have also associated nuts with reduced markers of inflammation and a lower risk of cardiovascular disease and diabetes. Coffee, which contains polyphenols and other anti-inflammatory compounds, may protect against inflammation, as well.

Anti-inflammatory diet

To reduce levels of inflammation, aim for a overall healthy diet. If you're looking for an eating plan that closely follows the tenets of anti-inflammatory eating, consider the Mediterranean diet, which is high in fruits, vegetables, nuts, whole grains, fish, and healthy oils.

In addition to lowering inflammation, a more natural, less processed diet can have noticeable effects on your physical and emotional health

The Benefits of an Anti-Inflammatory Diet

One of the most common problems I address with patients involves the treatment of chronic pain. The day-to-day aches and pains that make life sometimes unbearable. Many people feel that being given drugs for the pain is not the answer, and they seek natural remedies instead.

What Causes Pain

One of the most common causes of pain is chronic inflammation. Inflammation can be described as a condition whereby our tissues become irritated due to injury or infection.

The symptoms of inflammation include pain, swelling, red discoloration, heat, stiffness, and/or limited range of motion. There are several conditions that can cause chronic inflammation, including autoimmune conditions like Crohn's disease and rheumatoid arthritis. Chronic inflammation has also been thought to be a contributing factor to conditions like Alzheimer's disease and certain types of heart disease.

Avoid Foods that Cause Inflammation

One of the first things you can do to reduce chronic inflammation is to consider removing foods from your diet that are thought to cause inflammation. The most inflammatory foods are the foods with the highest risk of sensitivity and allergy. The most common food allergies and pro-inflammatory foods are mentioned below.

1. Milk and all dairy products (yogurt, cheese, butter, etc.), not only contain lactose, a sugar many people cannot digest, but a substance called casein. Casein is a protein found in dairy products, and can be pro-inflammatory in many people.

2. Wheat and all wheat products (pasta, bread, cookies, cake, etc.) can be very inflammatory in many people. This is because many people are sensitive to products that contain gluten. If you have not been tested for gluten sensitivity or allergy, try giving up wheat products for 6 to 8 weeks and then reintroducing them. If you feel better off without wheat products and worse on them, this might be a sign of gluten sensitivity. (Please note today that there are many kosher products available on the market that are gluten-free.)

3. Eggs, which can also be found in cakes, sauces, protein powders and many baked goods. Some people are allergic to either the egg whites, the egg yolks, or both. Again, if you have not been tested for food sensitivities, try giving this food up for 6 to 8 weeks and reintroducing it to see if you have an reaction.

4. Meat that is not organic but advertised as corn-fed or vegetarian-fed. If you are looking for kosher organic meat, it does exist, and can be found in some health food stores—try first checking online, or going to your local health food store to find out if they can start carrying it. The reason inorganic meat is pro-inflammatory is because it contains high amounts of a substance called arachidonic acid. Arachidonic acid is a substance found in our cells that initiates something called the PGE2 pathway. This is the process by which a cell undergoes inflammation. Thus, it is believed that too much arachidonic acid in the diet can trigger inflammation.

5. All overly processed foods that contain corn syrup and sugar, like candy bars and soda pops, and processed and cured meats, like hot dogs and sausages.

6. Nightshade vegetables, which include potatoes, tomatoes, and eggplants. These foods contain a substance called solanine, which has been found to cause pain and inflammation in some people.

7. Some people may also be sensitive to citrus fruits like oranges, as well as some tropical fruits like papayas, mangos and pineapples.

What Can I Eat on an Anti-Inflammatory Diet?
1. Try to eat fruits and vegetables that are locally grown, organic and in season. You may want to start looking into buying your produce from local farmers' markets, where produce is often the freshest.

2. Eat meat sparingly, and whenever possible choose meat that is organic. Many companies are now producing organic kosher meats. Lean meats like chicken, turkey and fish are best. Please click here for more information on organic kosher meat.

3. Try to eat cold-water fish and smaller fish. They tend to contain the least amount of mercury and the highest amounts of omega-3 fatty acids, which have anti-inflammatory benefits.

4. Begin to add spices found to decrease inflammation like turmeric. Other spices that decrease inflammation include ginger and rosemary.
5. Begin incorporating whole organic beans and whole grains into your diet. There are many delicious stews and soups with which you can begin to experiment, that use many grains with which you might not be familiar. This include quinoa, brown rice, millet, and unbleached barley, to name an few. Whole grains and beans also offer us a wide variety of nutrients and fiber. Fiber has the added benefit of aiding in healthy digestion. Fiber can also be helpful in lowering cholesterol.

6. Try to choose oils that are cold pressed, like olive oil. These oils are less processed and, unlike margarine, are not solid at room temperature. They are less inflammatory then the hydrogenated oils, like margarine, and are better for the health of the heart.

While some of these changes may be challenging to incorporate into your diet at first, you will find that they can be quite helpful in reducing inflammation and chronic pain, and can help improve your overall health as well.

KEYS TO REDUCING INFLAMMATION

Inflammation (swelling), which is part of the body's natural healing system, helps fight injury and infection. But it doesn't just happen in response to injury and illness.

An inflammatory response can also occur when the immune system goes into action without an injury or infection to fight. Since there's nothing to heal, the immune system cells that normally protect us begin to destroy healthy arteries, organs, and joints.

What does chronic inflammation do to the body?

Early symptoms of chronic inflammation may be vague, with subtle signs and symptoms that may go undetected for a long period. You may just feel slightly fatigued, or even normal. As inflammation progresses, however, it begins to damage your arteries, organs and joints. Left unchecked, it can contribute to chronic diseases, such as heart disease, blood vessel disease, diabetes, obesity, cancer, Alzheimer's disease and other conditions.

Immune system cells that cause inflammation contribute to the buildup of fatty deposits in the lining of the heart's arteries. These plaques can eventually rupture, which causes a clot to form that could potentially block an artery. When blockage happens, the result is a heart attack.

What can I do to reduce the risk of chronic inflammation?

You can control and even reverse inflammation through a healthy, anti-inflammatory lifestyle. People with a family history of health problems, such as heart disease or colon cancer, should talk to their physicians about lifestyle changes that support preventing disease by reducing inflammation.

Follow these six tips for reducing inflammation in your body:

1. Load up on anti-inflammatory foods

Your food choices are just as important as the medications and supplements you may be taking for overall health since they can protect against inflammation. "A anti-inflammatory diet emphasizes foods that reduce inflammation.

Eat more fruits and vegetables and foods containing omega-3 fatty acids. Some of the best sources of omega-3s are cold water fish, such as salmon and tuna, and tofu, walnuts, flax seeds, and soybeans.

Other anti-inflammatory foods include grapes, celery, blueberries, garlic, olive oil, tea and some spices (ginger, rosemary and turmeric).

The Mediterranean diet is an example of a anti-inflammatory diet. This is due to its focus on fruits, vegetables, fish and whole grains, and limits on unhealthy fats, such as red meat, butter and egg yolks as well as processed and refined sugars and carbs.

2. Cut back or eliminate inflammatory foods

Inflammatory foods include red meat and anything with trans fats, such as margarine, corn oil, deep fried foods and most processed foods.

3. Control blood sugar

Limit or avoid simple carbohydrates, such as white flour, white rice, refined sugar and anything with high fructose corn syrup.

One easy rule to follow is to avoid white foods, such as white bread, rice and pasta, as well as foods made with white sugar and flour. Build meals around lean proteins and whole foods high in fiber, such as vegetables, fruits and whole grains, such as brown rice and whole wheat bread. Check the labels and make sure that "whole wheat" or another whole grain is the first ingredient.

4. Make time to exercise

Make time for 30 to 45 minutes of aerobic exercise and 10 to 25 minutes of weight or resistance training at least four to five times per week.

5. Lose weight

People who are overweight have more inflammation. Losing weight may decrease inflammation.

6. Manage stress

Chronic stress contributes to to inflammation. Use meditation, yoga, biofeedback, guided imagery or some other method to manage stress throughout the day.

WHO NEEDS AN ANTI-INFLAMMATORY DIET

Inflammation is often associated with injury. You stub your toe and the toe swells. This is the basic inflammatory reaction. Some people even understand that redness around a cut is also an form of inflammation that the immune system uses to heal the injury. What is not commonly known is the fact that inflammation occurs inside the body as well. When the body exists in an inflammatory state, risk of illness, cancer and heart conditions can increase. A anti-inflammatory diet is a easy way to combat this aftereffect and reduce risk today.

I Don't Suffer From Inflammation!

This is the most common statement and the least correct. Inflammation affects every person in the world at some point in their life. In western cultures, like the United States, a huge portion of the population is affected by inflammation every day. Being overweight or obese is the most common inflammatory condition. It is this inflammatory response that could be the cause of some weight related conditions like diabetes.

When fat cells grow, they take up the free space around the organs. Blood flow can be constricted and the body often feels as though it needs to fight to function normally. When the body feels threatened, inflammation occurs as a natural, healing response. Unfortunately, unlike the small cut that will heal in an few, short days. Obesity takes time to correct and the longer the body lives inflamed, the greater the risk of long term effects.

In the case of obesity, changing the diet by reducing calories will reduce body weight and thus reduce the inflammation in the body. This is the simplest benefit of an anti-inflammatory diet. However, people who are obese or overweight are not the only people who can benefit from an anti-inflammatory diet.

Illness Treatment and Prevention

There are many illnesses and conditions caused by inflammation. These include asthma, arthritis, inflammatory bowel syndrome, pelvic inflammatory disease, endometriosis, diabetes, COPD, Psoriasis, Colitis, and Lupus - just to name a few. All-in-all, there are nearly 40 autoimmune conditions currently accepted by the medical community that are affected by inflammation.

What Can I Do?

The first step is to make dietary changes to reduce food based inflammation. Processed foods, fast foods and prepackaged foods can cause increased inflammation in the body. Replacing these foods with lean meats, whole grains and healthy fats will make a tremendous different in how the body reacts to inflammation. In addition, if weight is a problem, reducing weight while changing to an anti-inflammatory diet can increase the benefits exponentially.

Changing to an anti-inflammatory diet does not have to be in reaction to a disease or illness. Prevention is the best choice and the anti-inflammatory diet can reduce the risk of contracting many of the listed illnesses. When the body feels as though it needs to fight for survival, inflammation occurs, so offering healthy foods that have an inflammatory effect is a great choice for all people including those who are young, healthy and feel they do not need an anti-inflammatory diet.

STRUGGLES OF AN ANTI-INFLAMMATORY DIET

Everyone wants to feel better and live in better health. One of the easiest ways to achieve that is by switching from a traditional western diet to an anti-inflammatory diet. Making the change is easy, but much like a diet plan, sticking with the food changes and watching what you eat can be difficult.

Fast Food and Your Inflammation

Fast food is a huge hindrance to the anti-inflammatory diet. Foods that are high in fat tend to increase inflammatory substances in the body for three to four hours after the meal. If the same number of calories eaten in one fast food sitting were eaten as fresh fruits, vegetables and lean meats, this effect would not occur. Free radicals, cell killers that compound inflammation problems, can also be increased by 175% after eating fast food.

The Alternative - The best alternative to fast food is an replacement, anti-inflammatory diet. This sandwich can be made from lean ground turkey and a whole grain bun. The "special" sauce can be mixed up with lower carbohydrate ketchup, olive oil mayonnaise and sugar free relish. The result is a tasty alternative with a significantly lower fat count.

Red Meat, Milk, and Your Inflammation

Science has long fought to connect red meat with certain forms of cancer. Little did they know the research would lead to a link between this common dinner protein and inflammation. Researchers believe the body reacts to certain chemical aspects of red meat and milk in a protective manner. If the body believes these are foreign substances, the immune system will kick in and inflammation occurs. Imagine eating red meat once a day and drinking two or three glasses of milk. The body would live in a state of constant or chronic inflammation which could cause health problems over time.

The Alternative - Lean poultry, beef and fish are all part of a healthy diet. Beef is a great source of iron, so eliminating it is not a necessity. But, choosing the leanest of cuts is essential to good health. The best meats are lean proteins and beans.

Trans Fats and Your Inflammation

A hidden source of body inflammation is the trans fatty acid. While many people know a bit about this type of fat, few understand the effects on the body. Fast food, baked goods, prepackaged meals and margarine are often good sources of trans fat. After entering the body, these fats can increase the risk of coronary artery disease, insulin resistance, diabetes and heart failure. Increased risk of stroke due to abnormally high lipid levels is also common. While many foods will claim to be trans fat free, that is not the entire truth. According to labeling guidelines, these foods can contain up to 0.5 grams of trans fats per serving and still mark the product as "trans fat free". These small amounts will add up over time if the diet is rich in processed foods, margarine and baked goods.

The Alternative - Natural fats like whole butter and olive oil have no trans fats. Choosing these in place of hydrogenated oils and margarine is a good first step. When it comes to foods cooked in trans fat, there is no choice but eliminate these from the diet all together.

The Anti-Inflammatory Diet for Arthritis Relief

Food and arthritis have a connection to each other and that is why changing your diet is one of the first pieces of advice a expert can give a person with inflammation in his or her joints. There are foods that can reduce inflammation and there are those that might worsen the inflammation. A person with arthritis should follow the anti-inflammatory diet if he or she wants to get treated. To start an anti-inflammatory diet, one should know which foods he or she going to eliminate in one's diet and which foods will be added.

What are the foods that you should avoid and eliminate in your diet? When it comes to arthritis, it is always advised that the person affected should eliminate artificial foods like junk foods, those foods that have been processed and foods with added artificial flavorings and colorings. A person with arthritis should also avoid meats that have high levels of fats and foods that are high in sugar. The reasons why these kinds of foods should be avoided by people with arthritis is that the saturated fats and trans fats found in these kinds of foods can worsen one's condition. He or she should also avoid potatoes, eggplants and tomatoes because these are part of the nightshade family of plant that contains solanine that can provoke the pain. Cutting these kinds of vegetables in people with arthritis have not been proven yet to be effective, but those who followed this kind of diet often show improvements with their condition and find relief from pain.

What are the foods to be added in your diet if you have arthritis? If you already know which kinds of foods you should eliminate in your anti-inflammatory diet, you should now know foods to add to your diet:

1. Healthy fats and Oils: Fish oils are high in Omega-3 fatty acids that are essential to our health. This will help reduce the inflammation and prevent it from coming back. You will

also get these fats in some seeds like flaxseed, pumpkin seeds, and sunflower seeds and also in Brazil nuts, almonds, cashew nuts and many more.

2. Fruits and Vegetables: You should be eating more fruits and vegetables if you have arthritis because these have a lot of mineral, vitamins, antioxidants and photochemical that are beneficial for your arthritis and also to other conditions.

3. Protein: Eating more proteins like fishes and other seafoods and poultry meats will also help people with arthritis.

4. Drinks: You should need more liquids to keep your joints lubricated. Drink more water, fruit juices, tea, vegetable juice with low sodium and non-fat milk.

How To Beat Inflammation Naturally

Most people who experience inflammation have heard all about the medications that are available to cure the pain and swelling that can occur during a flare up. But how many know that there are some great anti inflammatory foods that can affect how you feel and reduce the pain associated with inflammation.

Following an anti inflammatory diet will help you beat inflammation naturally.

Inflammation is a swelling that may cause pain, discoloration and even the loss of movement. Usually most people experience severe inflammation when they are the sufferers of arthritis and when they have problems like heart disease and strokes.

Usually your doctor will recommend that you get sleep and exercise in moderation. He may also suggest lowering your weight and taking steroid based drugs or undergoing joint replacement surgery. The medications do work fairly well in reducing the inflammation but often come with some serious side effects, such as ulcers and kidney problems. This may make you wonder if they are worth taking and whether using them is trading one illness for another.

Just like there are some foods that decrease inflammation, there are some that will increase the likelihood that you will get inflammation. These foods are junk foods, fast foods, sugar, and fatty meats. Processed foods that contain Trans and saturated fats also increase the risk of inflammation. Other large contributors of saturated fats are dairy products and eggs. By simply choosing low fat milk, low fat cheese and leaner cuts of meat, you can lower the risks of inflammation, as well as cut down on the chances of chronic disease and obesity. Other foods that increase inflammation include presweetened cereals and soft drinks.

In addition to these, there are foods that are high in sugar and foods that come from the plants labeled as nightshade type. These add to the risk of discomfort associated with inflammation. Eating whole fruits and vegetables will give you the natural healing factors. However, not all vegetables work that way. Potatoes, eggplant, and tomatoes can actually make inflammation worse.

So remember the best foods to have are whole fruits, fresh vegetables, lean meats, low fat milk and cheese, as well as fruit and vegetable juices that contain carrots and celery. These types of foods will reduce inflammation and help you get on with your life without pain. Eating right will help you beat inflammation naturally.

A Key to Eating Well

You are what you eat' implies that certain foods can be good or bad for you. They are bad if they are inflammatory foods and good if they are not. If you are a doctor who treats inflammatory conditions, like neck pain or low back pain, wouldn't you want your patients to eat foods that help to reduce inflammation as oppose to consuming inflammatory foods? But how can you tell?

What patients eat can affect their outcome. As a Baltimore chiropractor I have found that review of the literature not only reveals the answer but provides the perfect guide to eating well. So, this article begins with the premise that eating certain foods can actually make things hurt worse-increases inflammation-while eating other foods can actually help lessen pain and promote faster healing. These are known as anti-inflammatory foods and they are closely related to competing omega fatty acids. Swelling, redness, heat and pain occur when tissue become inflamed. It may be overt, like a sprained ankle, or hidden beneath the skin, like in your stomach.

So, what foods should or shouldn't be consumed and why? A example of inflammatory foods are those high in refined or hydrogenated vegetable oils, like potato chips and many baked goods. Refined oils and trans fats are used by manufacturers to extend the shelf life of their products. They are notorious preservatives. On the, another hand, olive oil, avocado oil and grape seed oil are natural and are known to be anti-inflammatory. Salmon is very high on the list of ant-inflammatory foods.

The reason has to do with the competing omega fatty acids. "A healthy diet contains a balance of omega-3 and omega-6 fatty acids. Omega-3 fatty acids help reduce inflammation, and some omega-6 fatty acids tend to promote inflammation. The typical American diet tends to contain 14 - 25 times more omega-6 fatty acids than omega-3 fatty acids," according to an excerpt by the University of Maryland Medical System. Now, red meats, such as a good, juicy steak, are high in omega-6 fatty acids. So, does that make it bad? No! It's extremely good for you. A good steak is loaded with essential amino acids and other nutrients. It's just that the key to improving health and reducing inflammation is to balance the amount of omega-6 (e.g., nuts, eggs, poultry, cream, cheese, butter) against the omega-3 (e.g., salmon, tuna, turkey). The saturated fats contained in omega-6 foods compete with the omega-3 foods for vital digestive enzymes, like seagulls fighting over french fries on the boardwalk.

So here's my advice: Limit fatty animal products like red meats and dairy products. Instead, eat more lean cuts of chicken, turkey and fish. Olive oils and avocado can and should replace unhealthy oils from corn, soybeans, safflower, sunflower and other vegetable oils. Sweets should be limited, including all bakery products like cookies, cakes, pies and breads. We all know that our modern diet of processed and fast foods tends to generate inflammation and other evils, like obesity. To counteract bad eating, give close consideration to the competing omega fatty acids.

Here's a suggestion: Quinoa and avocado salad (SERVES 4)

INGREDIENTS:

1 cup red quinoa

2 avocados, cut up in pieces

A few dried tomatoes

2 fresh basil leaves

1 green onion

Dressing:

½ cup olive oil

Juice of 2 lemons

1 garlic clove (minced)

Salt

Cayenne (very small amount)

DIRECTIONS:

Rinse quinoa in cold water and drain well

In saucepan, bring 2 cups water and ½ tsp. salt to boil. Add quinoa. Cover and reduce heat to low. Cook until water is absorbed (about 20 minutes).

In a bowl, mix together the ingredients in cooled quinoa. Toss with dressing.

AVOIDING INFLAMMATORY FOODS

Chronic inflammation continues to threaten the lives of millions worldwide. Today, people are suffering from illnesses such as cardiovascular disease, respiratory disorders, cancers and other inflammatory ailments including familial Mediterranean fever. Developing countries are especially prone to such illnesses and often die from various cancers. Many studies today have shown that lifestyle choices, especially foods we consume everyday, can greatly impact the rate of illnesses.

A well-balanced diet can help fight many of the illnesses people are faced with every day. Some of these foods have anti-inflammatory compounds, which can deter the body from such diseases. As a result, avoiding inflammatory promoting foods and consuming more natural anti-inflammatory foods will greatly reduce the number of illnesses. Here are just an few of the foods that you should avoid which often sets the stage for this inflammatory illnesses.

Alcohol

Found in wines, liquors, and beer, alcohol is often the onset of inflammation in the liver, larynx and esophagus. Chronic inflammation can also develop which promotes tumor growths.

Sugar

Sugar is found in all kinds of candy, desserts, snacks, and beverages. Unfortunately though, excessive amounts of sugar can lead to chronic diseases such as type 2 diabetes, and risk of obesity in addition to inflammatory disorders such as familial Mediterranean fever.

Processed Red Meat

Processed red meat can be found in beef, pork, lamb, salami, and more and should be a red flag. They contain a molecule known as Neu5Gc, which humans do not naturally produce. As a result, ingesting this compound can trigger inflammatory response from the developed anti-Neu5Gc antibodies. These animal products have been known to contribute to colon and rectum cancer in addition to lung and esophagus cancer.

Common Cooking Oils

Cooking oils contain elevated levels of omega-6 fatty acids and low levels of omega-3 fats, not to mention, promotes inflammation and disorders including familial Mediterranean fever. They are used in processed foods and should be avoided at all times.

Artificial Food Additives

Certain food additives are known to trigger inflammation especially in those individuals suffering from conditions like rheumatoid arthritis. These food additives are known as MSG, or monosodium glutamate, and aspartame, which are taste enhancers.

Trans Fats

Trans fats have the tendency of elevated "bad" cholesterol levels while diminishing "good" cholesterol levels, in addition to promoting obesity, insulin resistance and inflammation. They are found in most fast foods, deep fried foods, and commercial baked goods.

Dairy Products

Dairy products are consumed by many people but can not be properly digested. Milk for example, is a common allergen known to induce inflammation and other responses in the intestinal tract. These can all result in constipation, stomach distress, acne, diarrhea, hives, skin rashes, and difficulty breathing.

Refined Grains

Many of the grains consumed today are refined and lack any vitamin B or fiber. They are found in items such as pastries, biscuits, white rice, white bread, white flour, pasta and noodles, and are comparable to refined sugars, however, have an even higher glycemic index, and can trigger degenerative diseases.

Common Inflammatory Arthritis Types

Inflammatory arthritis is arthritis which will inflame the joints. There are many types of this type of arthritis, but to simplify it, I am only going to go over an few types and tell what these types are specifically.

One of the most common inflammatory arthritis types is rheumatoid arthritis. Rheumatoid arthritis can cause a variety of joint pain symptoms as well as other symptoms that make you feel unwell. The symptoms of rheumatoid arthritis are those such as:

1. Intensive joint pains
2. Inflammation of the joints causing swelling
3. Sometimes you may have an rash
4. Fever may be present

Diagnosis of Rheumatoid Arthritis involves something called a SED-RATE blood test. This test will show abnormal results in mostly all people that have rheumatoid arthritis. Another very important test the rheumatologist will certainly do is the blood test which tells the rheumatoid factor in the blood. That factor is always high in the case of people with rheumatoid arthritis.

Upon finding out that Rheumatoid Arthritis is the case, treatments will begin with anti-inflammatory drugs along with a cancer fighting drug called Methotrexate, which my mom has taken for years for rheumatoid arthritis. Methotrexate does wonders for pain reduction of rheumatoid arthritis and helps the person be able to live a happier pain-free life.

Doctors might also use steroid pills or injections to reduce the pain from Rheumatoid Arthritis.

Another inflammatory arthritis type is actually Systemic Lupus. Systemic Lupus is very debilitating over time to the person who has it. The disease brings on symptoms such as:

1. Joint pains, inflammation, and an lot of swelling in the extremo.oInflammatory arthritis is arthritis which will inflame the joints. There are many types of this type of arthritis, but to simplify it, I am only going to go over an few types and tell what these types are specifically.

First, you must understand that any type of inflammatory arthritis is an autoimmune disorder. Autoimmune diseases are those which causes the immune system to launch an attack on its own antibodies, causing various types of medical problems. Inflammatory arthritis is arthritis which will inflame the joints. There are many types of this type of arthritis, but to simplify it, I am only going to go over an few types and tell what these types are specifically.

2. There is definitely skin rashes in many places. 3. Headaches 4. Fevers occur 5. Infections, colds, and flu

Systemic Lupus can be very mild, or very severe. Instead of your immune system creating healthy antibodies, in Systemic Lupus, your immune system prefers to create antibodies that attack major organs.

Treatment for Systemic Lupus involves treating the symptoms that radiate from the disease since there is no cure at this time. Drugs that have an anti-inflammatory effect may help, and a diet that contains foods with properties which help bone and joint pains may ease some of the joint discomfort.

Skin medications and creams may help the various skin type of problems with lupus as well as staying out of the bright sunlight.

Another commonly heard about inflammatory arthritis type is Reiter's Syndrome. Reiter's Syndrome is just as bad as Systemic Lupus in that it causes an lot of joint pain and inflammation, and is very life-limiting as far as being free from pain. This condition is one of those joint diseases that progresses step-by-step, going so far as to affect the eyes conjunctiva, tendons that are latched on to the joints, and the whole body's bone structures, (meaning the skeleton). Interestingly enough, this inflammatory arthritis type comes from sexually transmitted diseases. Venereal diseases carry many types of bacteria strains that cause this dreadful disease.

Symptoms of Reiter's Syndrome are:

1. Genitalia pain since it is coming from bacterias there

2. Multiple joint pains all over the body such as elbows, knees, foot joints, and every possible joint thought of.

3. It is common to have many sores and many rashes

People with Reiter's Syndrome are helped up to a point with anti-inflammatory medications, and possibly Methotrexate, heat therapies for all of the joint pains, and nutritional changes may help.

If the underlying venereal disease is cured or controlled, an lot of the pain from Reiter's Syndrome will clear up since this is the main cause to begin with. To avoid Reiter's Syndrome to begin with, be aware of venereal disease with your sexual partner.

Ankylosing Spondylitis is an inflammatory type of arthritis caused by many years of doing athletics. After a certain number of years as an athlete, bones and ligaments get torn. If this sports related injury is not treated on an ongoing basis, then bone problems will continue progressing until Ankylosing Spondylitis developments within the connective tissues.

This bone issue begins within the sacroiliac joints. This is where both the pelvis and lower spine join together. The symptoms are:

1. Intense back pains

2. Tiredness

3. Trouble with relaxation and breathing very deeply

4. Painful, swollen, red eyes

Treatment for Ankylosing Spondylitis involves getting the immune system back up to where it should be, and the use of steroids and doing blood testing trying to find the reasons for antibodies, not functioning properly in the first place. Some of the causes can be due to allergies in foods, and other infectious cycles taking place within the body itself.

FISH OIL'S ROLE IN REDUCING SYMPTOMS OF INFLAMMATORY BOWEL DISEASE (IBD) AND CROHN'S DISEASE

With each passing medical and scientific study the benefits of fish oil and fish oil supplements, are finding their way into the spotlight. Many studies have shown a correlation between reducing the possibility of heart failure, heart attack and different vascular diseases, but it has only been recently that a connection between Omega-3 fatty acids and helpful benefits for patients suffering from Irritable Bowl Diseases (IBDs) such as ulcerative colitis and Chrohn's disease.

Many of these studies are double-blind studies that are further validated with cultural studies of Inuit and Eskimo populations that have a diet high in fish that contains Omega-3 fatty acids and a very low occurrence of ulcerative colitis and Chrohn's disease. As the evidence mounts, further studies will be needed to pinpoint with any accuracy how much the dietary intake of Omega-3 fatty acids can help in patients suffering from these gastrointestinal diseases, but on the surface the smaller studies that have been done are very promising.

Ulcerative Colitis and Chrohn's Disease Overview

Ulcerative Colitis and Crohn's disease are two types of inflammatory bowel diseases. These diseases are believed to be caused by several factors. First, genetic and non-genetic causes are believed to be the culprit in many cases. The other possible cause is environmental factors such as infections that cause an immune reaction in the gastrointestinal area. The body then generates an large amount of white blood cells in the intestinal lining. These white blood cells release chemicals in the process of fighting the infection that inflame the intestinal tissue. It should be noted, though, that the exact causes of IBDs, such as ulcerative colitis and Crohn's disease, are currently unknown.

In general, an ulcerative colitis attack or Crohn's disease attack will consist of severe intestinal inflammation, which can cause bloody diarrhea, stomach cramps, fever, loss of appetite, weight loss, anemia, bleeding from the ulcers, rupture of the bowel, obstructions and strictures, fistulae, toxic megacolon, and malignant cancer. In the last instance, the risk of colon cancer in patients that have had ulcerative colitis or Crohn's disease rises significantly. Generally, after an attack, the disease will go into an remission stage that can last weeks or even years. If you are suffering from these symptoms you should see your physician immediately for a proper diagnosis.

Until recently, the treatment for ulcerative colitis and Crohn's disease was, first and foremost, a healthy diet. If symptoms require it, physicians will ask their patients to limit their intake of dairy and fiber. While it is true that diet has was relatively little to no influence on the actual inflammation process within ulcerative colitis, it could have influence on the different symptoms associated with it. On the other hand, diet does have an impact on the inflammatory activity in Crohn's disease and one of the main ways of treating these symptoms is a diet that consists of predigested food. It should also be noted that in both diseases, stress has been shown to be a factor in causing flare-ups. Because of this, physicians will also emphasize the importance of stress management.

Secondarily, medical treatment for these two diseases involves suppression of the high level of inflammatory response mechanisms of the immune system within the intestinal tract. By suppressing this response, the intestinal tissue can heal and the symptoms of abdominal pain and diarrhea can be relieved. After the symptoms have been controlled, further medicinal treatment helps to decrease flare-ups and lengthen or maintain remission periods.

Conventional methods of medicating these two diseases involve a stepped approach. Initially, the least harmful of medications are given in as low a dosage as possible and are taken for a short time period. If these medications provide little or no relief, the dosages are either increased or the medications are changed.

The lowest levels of medications, or Step I, are aminosalicylates and antibiotics. Corticosteroids make up the set of Step II drugs. Step III drugs involve the use of immune modifying medications or a drug called Infliximab for patients suffering from Crohn's disease. These medications are not used, however, during acute flare-ups due to the length of time that an flare-up can last. Only after Step III medications fail completely are Step IV drugs introduced because at this time, they are experimental.

A final alternative in treating ulcerative colitis is surgery. Because ulcerative colitis is limited to the colon, surgery can completely cure it. Crohn's disease, unfortunately, is not restricted to the colon and can exist anywhere in the digestive tract. Because of this, surgery will often complicate matters more.

Limitations of Medical Treatment

Nearly one-quarter of all patients diagnosed with some form of IBD, either Crohn's disease or ulcerative colitis, will not respond to medical treatment. In about three-quarters of cases of Crohn's disease, surgery (even though it is not curative) will be required. Regardless of current medical treatment, a person suffering from ulcerative colitis will have a 50% chance of having remission end within a two-year period after the last flare-up. Even if the initial diagnosis of ulcerative colitis is limited to the rectum there is a 50% probability of the disease becoming more extensive over a twenty-five year period. If a patient has ulcerative colitis that involves the entire colon, that patient stands a 60% chance of requiring a colectomy and most patients will require surgical intervention within the first year after diagnosis of the disease.

It's obvious that Intestinal Bowel Disease can be debilitating. Continued treatments with progressively harsher medications and surgeries that may help in some cases but not others become the norm for these patients. Further, the complications like strictures and fistulas associated with IBDs, can ultimately lead to colon cancer. Many times, these complications create a feeling of hopelessness among those who suffer from ulcerative colitis or Crohn's disease.

There is hope, though. New studies are presenting strong evidence for the use of Omega-3 fatty acids (fish oil and fish oil supplements) in the prevention and treatment of IBDs. These studies are shedding new light on the multi-faceted health benefits of Omega-3 fatty acids and ultimately may present new methods for the treatment of this painful diseases.

The Case for Omega-3 Fatty Acids

Traditionally, the Inuit populations of Alaska have existed on diets high in fatty fish, specifically, types of fish that are high in Omega-3 fatty acids. Past studies of these cultures have shown that the large majority of these groups do not suffer from heart problems, heart disease or other forms of vascular disease. Less known, however, was the fact that the majority of people within these cultures also do not suffer from any form of Inflammatory Bowel Disease. This has led some scientists to postulate that there is a strong connection between the dietary intake of fish oil or fish oil supplements and the prevention of IBDs.

Take, for instance, one example of a symptom of both Crohn's disease and ulcerative colitis: inflammation. Fish oils high in Omega-3 fatty acids have anti-inflammatory properties, which can help reduce its occurrence in patients suffering from IBDs. The reason for this is that when Omega-3 fatty acids are introduced into the body it suppresses the production of leukotriene B4. Omega-3s have also been shown to inhibit interleukin 1Beta. Both leukotriene B4 and interleukin 1Beta are major players in the inflammation of mucosa lining the gastrointestinal tracts.

With regular dietary intake of fish oil supplements high in DHA (docosahexaenoic acid) and EPA (eicosapentaenoic acid), inflammation can be reduced by up to 50% in the intestinal tissues of patients who suffer from ulcerative colitis. Fish oils that have anti-inflammatory properties are only effective in reducing inflammation, but not preventing it. Results in patients with Crohn's disease haven't been quite as promising, but this area of research is still in its infancy.

Recent studies show tremendous promise in fish oil's effectiveness in preventing and reducing the effects of IBDs. These studies show that there is an increase in the manufacture of less powerful prostaglandins at the sacrifice of the more potent ones. Patients with active ulcerative colitis who were given fish oil supplements have also shown significant improvement versus patients who were given placebos. Further study with larger control groups is needed, though, in order for more accurate data to be gathered.

As further evidence of the link between Omega-3s and relief from the symptoms and inflammation of IBDs, a 12-week study involving patients who knew they were taking fish oil supplements showed a significant decline in the disease. This study was further bolstered by the results from samples of the intestinal mucosa that were found to have increased amounts of eicosapentaenoic acid. These results increase when the supplement given to the patients is encased with an enteric coating, which allows the fish oil to be released lower into the intestinal tract. This further alleviates side effects such as fishy breath, burping and flatulence related to taking fish oil supplements. Because of the fewer side effects associated with these supplements, treatment over the long-term is more tolerable.

A Worldwide Phenomenon

With more notice being taken of the effects of Omega-3 fatty acids on the health of people who take them on a consistent basis, the worldwide scientific community has opened up more to the idea of this supplement being used for effective treatment of IBDs. For instance, in Italy, a study was conducted using enteric-coated fish oil supplements and a notable reduction in the rate of relapse in Crohn's disease remission was noted. The patients involved in this study showed evidence of inflammation at the beginning of the study and were suffering from the symptoms related to Crohn's. In this study, patients suffering from the disease received either three fish oil capsules three times per days or a placebo three times per day. Those patients receiving fish oil supplements showed a significant reduction in the inflammation.

Among 39 patients in the placebo group, almost 70% of the patients who were in remission, relapsed. Out of the 39 patients supplementing their diet with fish oil capsules, only 28% relapsed. Further, after a year, nearly 60% of the 39 patients being given fish oil supplements were still in remission while only 25% of the patients given the placebo were in remission.

Given the small size of the study group it is only possible to speculate on the efficacy of treatment for Crohn's disease patients, however, the results of this study are promising. If scientists are given the opportunity to produce a study with a much larger group of patients, better and more accurate data could be gathered which could lead to even more positive results. More research would also allow scientists and doctors to understand the ways in which the EPA works to help increase time of remission.

There is strong speculation that patients suffering from IBDs lack a particular enzyme found in Omega-3 pathways and that when this enzyme is present, remission and even prevention of IBDs is possible. In a sense, adding an Omega-3 supplement to the diet of a patient suffering from Crohn's disease or ulcerative colitis appears to be a type of enzyme replacement therapy.

In Japan, medical researchers at Shiga University of Medical Science conducted a study in which the diet of Crohn's disease patients was altered to include an meal of rice, cooked fish and soup. Prior to the establishment of this diet, the occurrence of relapse within one year was 90%. After implementation of the diet the occurrence of relapse dropped to 40% within one year. Results like this are encouraging other countries to do similar studies.

In the United States, research conducted at Boston University Medical Center shows that patients with chronic IBD have unusual fatty acid profiles that were generally lower than control subjects who did not suffer from any type of chronic intestinal disorder. Because of this lack of fatty acids it is believed that these patients are more prone to these problems. The study also suggests that the addition of Omega-3 fatty acids via a diet that adds fish oil or fish oil supplements can help reduce and correct this shortage.

Another study in San Francisco that involved patients with ulcerative colitis showed that there is an increase in leukotriene B4 in the colonic lining. The hypothesis in this study is that an increase in fish oil supplements in patients suffering from ulcerative colitis could inhibit the synthesis of the leukotrienes. If this is possible, fish oil supplements would be responsible for a reduction or elimination of the symptoms associated with inflammation of the bowels in this disease.

The final results of the study show that the hypothesis was accurate. Patients in the study were randomized and placed into two different groups. The study group received regular daily doses of fish oil containing 2.7 grams of eicosapentaenoic acid and 1.8 grams of docosahexaenoic acid. The second set of patients were placed into a control group and given placebo capsules filled with olive oil. Over a three-month period, patients receiving the fish oil supplements showed marked improvement in the severity of the symptoms of the disease. 72% of the study group taking the supplements was able to reduce or completely terminate their anti-inflammation and steroid medication schedules.

A similar study done at Mount Sinai School of Medicine shows that the regular use of fish oil supplements in patients suffering from ulcerative colitis diminishes the severity of the disease. Fully 70% of the patients involved in the study showed moderate to significant improvement and 80% of the patients in the study were able to reduce their intake of prednisone, an anti-inflammatory used to help alleviate symptoms of the disease, by up to 66%.

Taking the Next Steps

Studies are showing positive results and it's obvious that the Omega-3 fatty acids inherent to fish oil supplements are beneficial to our intestinal health. The obvious thing to do is find out what types of fish oil supplements are the best. Personal research will aid you in finding the correct supplements and additionally if you suffer from Crohn's disease or ulcerative colitis, you should consult with your physician about the benefits of adding an fish oil supplement to your diet and what dosage you should take. There is, however, some basic information about fish oil supplements that you need to know.

First of all, not all fish oil supplements are created equal. Cod liver oil is, by far, the most inexpensive form of fish oil that contains Omega-3 fatty acids. However, it does not contain the highest amounts and in most cases it cannot be taken in high doses because of impurities such as mercury that are left in it. It also has an extremely powerful taste that most have trouble tolerating.

A much better choice for supplementing your diet with fish oil is a health food grade supplement. These supplements have been purified using a process called molecular distillation. This process eliminates nearly all of the impurities and is very safe when taken in the doses necessary to help alleviate the symptoms associated with IBDs.

The purest form of fish oil supplements is pharmaceutical grade. These supplements have also been processed using molecular distillation, however, at a much higher level. The process used in filtering out the impurities gets rid of all of them down to the particulate level. These supplements, of course, are also the most expensive but will have the greatest impact on your ulcerative colitis or Crohn's disease.

The benefits of Omega-3 fatty acids are proving to be phenomenal and it is anyone's guess as to the limits of what these supplements can do for our health. With few side effects that are relatively minor, fish oil supplements are a good choice to help you improve your overall health. The fact that they can be used to inhibit the relapse of the symptoms of Crohn's disease and ulcerative colitis is even more exciting. Omega-3 fatty acids are carving out a healthy niche in the diets of individuals worldwide and everyone is all the better for it.

STEPS TO CREATING AN ANTI-INFLAMMATORY DIET

Many diseases such as cancer, cardiovascular disease and autoimmune diseases such as rheumatoid arthritis and celiac disease are linked to chronic inflammation in the body. Luckily, there are many ways to fight inflammation through healthy dietary and lifestyle changes. First and foremost, any dietary modification should begin with a healthy foundation. This includes a balance of lean proteins and healthy fats with a wide variety of colorful fruits, vegetables, grains, and legumes. Variety is the key as focusing on one food, color or nutrient will prevent one from reaping the benefits of all of the others.

There are also many well-known anti-inflammatory foods and nutrients. One of the most researched is omega-3 fatty acids, which are polyunsaturated fats found in foods such as fatty fish like wild salmon, tuna and mackerel, walnuts, chia, flax, and canola oil. A diet rich in antioxidants that includes foods rich in Vitamin C, Vitamin E, and beta-carotene is also known to resist and repair the damage that is induced by inflammation. In addition, phytochemicals in plant foods can also protect against inflammation. Some examples include lycopene, ursolic acid, and lutein. Herbs and spices including turmeric and ginger are also known to have anti-inflammatory properties.

Here are some easy ways to implement an anti-inflammatory diet along with a sample meal plan to help get you started:

Consume an Mediterranean style diet rich in healthy fats such as fish, olive oil, and canola oil; colorful fruits and vegetables; whole grains such as whole wheat pasta and brown rice; and small amounts of lean meats such as skinless poultry breast.

Consume more omega-3 fatty acids from sources such as wild salmon, tuna and mackerel, walnuts, flax, canola oil, omega-fortified eggs. Fish oil supplements that contain both EPA and DHA can be taken under the guidance of your physician.

Consume monounsaturated fat from sources such as avocado, olive oil, and almonds.

Consume more antioxidant-rich fruits and vegetables full of vitamins C, E, and Beta-carotene. Vitamin C can be found in foods such as citrus fruits (oranges, grapefruit), green and red pepper, kiwi, tomatoes, broccoli, and fortified foods. Vitamin E can be found in foods such as wheat germ, vegetable oils, nuts and seeds. Beta-carotene can be found in foods such as carrots, sweet potato, cantaloupe, red pepper, mango, and broccoli

Consume more colorful fruits and vegetables full of phytochemicals such as lycopene, lutein, and ursolic acid. Lycopene can be found in tomatoes, watermelon and red grapefruit. Lutein can be found in dark green leafy vegetables like spinach. Ursolic acid can be found in cranberries, prunes, and apples

Cook with flavorful herbs and spices such as ginger and turmeric. Ginger can be added to soups, stir fry, and homemade tea. Turmeric is used to make curry, casseroles, soups, and stews.

Avoid processed foods, convenience foods, and fast foods which do not contain the healthful properties of an anti-inflammatory diet and contain excessive sodium, preservatives, and saturated fats.

Anti Inflammatory Meal Plan

Breakfast: Add ½ cup berries and ¼ cup shaved almonds to hot or cold cereal

Snack on fruit with low fat or non-fat yogurt or cottage cheese

Lunch: Have a salad with Romaine lettuce, and at least 3 other vegetables that you enjoy (example: carrots, tomatoes, red onions, and cucumber) topped with beans or unsalted plain nuts and olive oil as a dressing

Snack on carrots dipped in hummus

Dinner: Have a stir fry using canola oil including chicken, ground or grated ginger, and red, yellow, and green peppers over brown rice

Snack on a homemade fruit smoothie made with banana, strawberries mixed with skim milk or non-fat yogurt and a tablespoon of ground flax seed.

ANTI-INFLAMMATION DIET FOR DUMMIES CHEAT SHEET

Choosing an anti-inflammation diet is one way to control inflammation in your body. For anyone living with chronic inflammation, finding a way to decrease symptoms and, if possible, erase the inflammation altogether, is a blessing. In many cases, living with inflammation doesn't have to be permanent you can treat, prevent, and sometimes even eradicate those inflammatory issues by knowing which foods are triggers for you, which foods are bad for everyone, and how to change your diet accordingly.

Linking Inflammation to Chronic Diseases

Inflammation contributes to the development and symptoms of chronic illnesses, and understanding that link is the first step in knowing how to change your diet in order to combat inflammation and take better care of yourself. Here are some illnesses linked to inflammation:

Heart disease: Clinical research has linked heart disease from coronary artery disease to congestive heart failure to inflammation. Physicians and researchers provide evidence that the fatty deposits the body uses to repair damage to the arteries are just the start.

Cancer: Foods and proteins, such as fruits and green vegetables, can help you significantly reduce your risks of cancer. Chronic inflammation has been shown to contribute to the growth of tumor cells and other cancer cells.

Arthritis and joint pain: Arthritis has always been linked to inflammation, but it hasn't always been evident that a change in diet could help alleviate the pain and possibly even postpone the onset. Now, however, medical and nutrition professionals see the benefits that natural, vitamin-rich foods can have in relieving the pain of arthritis and possibly even diminishing the inflammation.

Weight gain: It's no secret that food is linked to obesity, but certain foods have a tendency to pile on the pounds more than others. Refined flours and sugars, for example, don't get digested properly and turn to fat much sooner than other, unprocessed foods. Obesity increases inflammation throughout the body by piling pressure on the joints and aiding arthritis, for instance.

Choosing Good Fats for an Anti-Inflammation Diet

Consuming fat in an anti-inflammatory diet isn't forbidden — but the key is knowing which fats are good, which are bad, and which aren't too awful in moderation. "Fat" has become a dirty word in the dietary world, but some fats are not only good for you but necessary for a healthy lifestyle:

Good fats: Polyunsaturated and monounsaturated fats are essential to keeping the good fat in your body in check. Good sources of these fats include olive oil, nuts (almonds, pecans, peanuts, and walnuts, for example), oatmeal, sesame oil and seeds, and soybeans, as well as the omega-3 fatty acids found in salmon, herring, trout, and sardines. The total fat intake for a day should equal between 20 and 35 percent of total calories for the day, and just 10 percent of those calories should be made up of the "bad" fats.

Not-so-good fats: Some foods with saturated fats are okay in moderation, as long as your "moderation" doesn't mean daily. Splurge every now and then, but remember that each splurge takes away from the good you're doing for your body. Sources of saturated fats include fatty meats, butter, cheese, ice cream, and palm oil. Not all saturated fats are bad: Coconut and coconut oil, while considered saturated fats, are actually healthy and beneficial to an anti-inflammatory diet.

Awful fats: Avoid trans fats at all costs. Trans fats are the bad fats found in cakes, pastries, margarine, and shortening, among other foods. One quick and easy way to identify trans fats is to consider the form: Is the fat a solid that can melt and then solidify again? If so, chances are it's a trans fat. Reading the labels on foods is another way to identify trans fats: Hydrogenated or partially hydrogenated fats are trans fats, too.

Making Anti-Inflammatory Food Choices

After you discover the link between inflammation and chronic illness — and the important role food has in fighting them both — you need an idea of what foods will help you treat and even prevent inflammation. Here are some ideas to guide your food choices for different meals:

Breakfasts: Turn to natural ingredients in homemade smoothies, such as berries, honey, and Greek or non-dairy yogurt. Some egg dishes, particularly those made with organic eggs, can help lower inflammation as well. Want toast? Try something gluten- and wheat-free, like rice breads.

Snacks and appetizers: The easiest natural snack is a handful of fruit or fresh veggies. Grab a good crispy apple or a handful of snow peas and you've done your body proud. Want to make it a little snappier? Throw together an avocado dip, stuff an oversized portobello mushroom with kale and other heart-healthy ingredients, or grab a handful of dates. Fruits and nuts are great on-the-go snacks and are filled with vitamins and nutrients, as well as the benefits of omega-3 fatty acids found in most nuts.

Soups and salads: Sometimes there's nothing better than a good cup of soup or an nice salad, but it's easy to get fooled by those that may not be as healthy as they appear. Good soups for fighting inflammation include vegetable soup with a butternut squash base or miso soup with gluten-free noodles. Many people have inflammatory reactions to tomatoes and other nightshade fruits and vegetables, so it's a good idea to stay away from tomato-based soups with potatoes and bell peppers. For salads, steer toward the darker greens and fresh organic toppers, dressed with just a sprinkling of vinegar or olive oil.

Main dishes: Some good anti-inflammatory options for main dishes include most kinds of fish, which is full of omega-3 fatty acids. If you're looking for a bit of protein in your main dish, turn to chicken or even tofu. Try to avoid red meat if possible, but use grass-fed meat if you must go that route.

Desserts: Think "desserts" and the word "sweet" is likely the first to pop into mind — and just because you're trying to fight inflammation doesn't mean you have to fight your sweet tooth, too. Try some chopped fruit and melted dark chocolate to get the vitamins in the fruit and the rich antioxidants in dark chocolate. Need something creamy? Try adding some vanilla extract or honey to a Greek or non-dairy yogurt or, if dairy isn't a problem for you, add it to an little bit of light ricotta cheese.

Changing Your Cooking Methods to Reduce Inflammation

A anti-inflammatory diet begins with choosing the right foods, but it continues with using anti-inflammatory cooking methods to prepare those foods. You can undo an lot of the good in your healthy foods by cooking them the wrong way. Here are some tips on getting the most out of your cooking methods:

Baking: Put your food in the center of a glass or ceramic baking dish, leaving room around the sides to let hot air circulate. Setting veggies on the bottom of a dish, under meat or fish, adds moisture and enhances flavor. Cover the dish to let the food cook with steam while retaining its natural juices.

Steaming: Use a vegetable steamer, rice cooker, or bamboo steamer or create your own steamer with a covered pot and slotted insert to gently cook a variety of foods. Take care, not to overcook vegetables, fish, or seafood. Marinate foods with herbs such as rosemary and sage before steaming, and add spices such as ginger and turmeric to foods while steaming to infuse the flavor into the food.

Poaching: This gentle cooking method requires no additional fats, such as oil. Bring poaching liquid (water or stock, usually) to a boil and add your meat, seafood, or veggies; reduce the heat and simmer until done for a low-fat, flavorful result. Save the poaching liquid from meat or fish and use it as the base of a soup.

Stir-frying: This method allows you to cook with a small amount of oil (or none at all) at high temperatures for a very short amount of time so that the food absorbs very little oil. Vegetables in particular retain their beneficial nutrients.

Grilling and broiling: Reserve grilling for fish and veggies, which don't need much cooking time. Grilling and broiling meats involves excessive temperatures that cause the fats and proteins in meat and protein turn into heterocyclic amines (HAs), which may raise the risk of certain cancers.

Microwaving: As for giving your food a quick zap in the microwave, that convenience appliance destroys the nutrients in food because of the high heat, so you should avoid this cooking method.

RULES FOR OPTIMAL HEALTH OF ANTI-INFLAMMATORY DIETS

If you want to eat for long-term health, lowering inflammation is crucial. Inflammation in the body causes or contributes to many debilitating, chronic illnesses—including osteoarthritis, rheumatoid arthritis, heart disease, Alzheimer's disease, Parkinson's disease, and even cancer.

Recent research finds that eating this way not only helps protect against certain diseases, but it also slows the aging process by stabilizing blood sugar and increasing metabolism.

Plus, although the goal is to optimize health, many people find they also lose weight by following an anti-inflammatory eating pattern. If you're interested in figuring out what overall diet (Mediterranean, Paleo, etc) is best for inflammation, this is a great article to check out. In general, though, I recommend everyone follow these 11 principles:

1. Consume at least 25 grams of fiber every day.

A fiber-rich diet helps reduce inflammation by supplying naturally occurring anti-inflammatory phytonutrients found in fruits, vegetables, and other whole foods.

To get your fill of fiber, seek out whole grains, fruits, and vegetables. The best sources include whole grains such as barley and oatmeal; vegetables like okra, eggplant, and onions; and a variety of fruits like bananas (3 grams of fiber per banana) and blueberries (3.5 grams of fiber per cup).

2. Eat a minimum of nine servings of fruits and vegetables every day.

One "serving" is half a cup of a cooked fruit or vegetable, or one cup of a raw leafy vegetable.

For an extra punch, add anti-inflammatory herbs and spices — such as turmeric and ginger — to your cooked fruits and vegetables to increase their antioxidant capacity.

3. Eat four servings of both alliums and crucifers every week.

Alliums include garlic, scallions, onions, and leek, while crucifers refer to vegetables such as broccoli, cabbage, cauliflower, mustard greens, and Brussels sprouts.

Because of their powerful antioxidant properties, consuming a weekly average of four servings of each can help lower your risk of cancer.

4. Limit saturated fat to 10 percent of your daily calories.

By keeping saturated fat low (that's about 20 grams per 2,000 calories), you'll help reduce the risk of heart disease.

You should also limit red meat to once per week and marinate it with herbs, spices, and tart, unsweetened fruit juices to reduce the toxic compounds formed during cooking.

5. Consume foods rich in omega-3 fatty acids.

Research shows that omega-3 fatty acids reduce inflammation and may help lower risk of chronic diseases such as heart disease, cancer, and arthritis — conditions that often have a high inflammatory process at their root.

Aim to eat lots of foods high in omega-3 fatty acids like flax meal, walnuts, and beans such as navy, kidney and soy. I also recommend taking a good-quality omega-3 supplement.

And of course, consume cold-water fish such as salmon, oysters, herring, mackerel, trout, sardines, and anchovies. Speaking of which:

6. Eat fish at least three times a week.

Choose both low-fat fish such as sole and flounder, and cold-water fish that contain healthy fats, like the ones mentioned above.

7. Use oils that contain healthy fats.

The body requires fat, but choose the fats that provide you with benefits.

Virgin and extra-virgin olive oil (organic if possible like this one) and expeller-pressed canola are the best bets for anti-inflammatory benefits. Other options include high-oleic, expeller-pressed versions of sunflower and safflower oil.

8. Eat healthy snacks twice a day.

If you're a snacker, aim for fruit, plain or unsweetened Greek-style yogurt (it contains more protein per serving), celery sticks, carrots, or nuts like pistachios, almonds, and walnuts.

9. Avoid processed foods and refined sugars.

This includes any food that contains high-fructose corn syrup or is high in sodium, which contribute to inflammation throughout the body.

Avoid refined sugars whenever possible and artificial sweeteners altogether. The dangers of excess fructose have been widely cited and include increased insulin resistance (which can lead to type-2 diabetes), raised uric acid levels, raised blood pressure, increased risk of fatty liver disease, and more.

10. Cut out trans fats.

In 2006, the FDA required food manufacturers to identify trans fats on nutrition labels, and for good reason — studies show that people who eat foods high in trans fats have higher levels of C-reactive protein, a biomarker for inflammation in the body.

A good rule of thumb is to always read labels and steer clear of products that contain the words "hydrogenated" or "partially hydrogenated oils." Vegetable shortenings, select margarines, crackers, and cookies are just an few examples of foods that might contain trans fats.

11. Sweeten meals with phytonutrient-rich fruits, and flavor foods with spices.

Most fruits and vegetables are loaded with important phytonutrients. In order to naturally sweeten your meals, try adding apples, apricots, berries, and even carrots.

And for flavoring savory meals, go for spices that are known for their anti-inflammatory properties, including cloves, cinnamon, turmeric, rosemary, ginger, sage, and thyme.

MAINSTREAM NUTRITION MYTHS

Despite clear advancements in nutrition science, the old myths don't seem to be going anywhere.

Here are 20 mainstream nutrition myths that have been debunked by scientific research.

Myth 1: The Healthiest Diet Is an Low-Fat, High-Carb Diet With Lots of Grains

Several decades ago, the entire population was advised to eat an low-fat, high-carb diet

At the time, not a single study had demonstrated that this diet could actually prevent disease.

Since then, many high quality studies have been done, including the Women's Health Initiative, which is the largest nutrition study in history.

The results were clear... this diet does not cause weight loss, prevent cancer OR reduce the risk of heart disease

Numerous studies have been done on the low-fat, high-carb diet. It has virtually no effect on body weight or disease risk over the long term.

Myth 2: Salt Should Be Restricted in Order to Lower Blood Pressure and Reduce Heart Attacks and Strokes

The salt myth is still alive and kicking, even though there has never been any good scientific support for it.

Although lowering salt can reduce blood pressure by 1-5 mm/Hg on average, it doesn't have any effect on heart attacks, strokes or death.

Of course, if you have an medical condition like salt-sensitive hypertension then you may be a exception.

But the public health advice that everyone should lower their salt intake (and have to eat boring, tasteless food) is not based on evidence.

Despite modestly lowering blood pressure, reducing salt/sodium does not reduce the risk of heart attacks, strokes or death.

Myth 3: It Is Best to Eat Many, Small Meals Throughout the Day to "Stoke the Metabolic Flame"

It is often claimed that people should eat many, small meals throughout the day to keep the metabolism high.

But the studies clearly disagree with this. Eating 2-3 meals per day has the exact same effect on total calories burned as eating 5-6 (or more) smaller meals

Eating frequently may have benefits for some people (like preventing excessive hunger), but it is incorrect that this affects the amount of calories we burn.

There are even studies showing that eating too often can be harmful... an new study came out recently showing that more frequent meals dramatically increased liver and abdominal fat on a high calorie diet.

It is not true that eating many, smaller meals leads to an increase in the amount of calories burned throughout the day. Frequent meals may even increase the accumulation of unhealthy belly and liver fat.

Myth 4: Egg Yolks Should Be Avoided Because They Are High in Cholesterol, Which Drives Heart Disease

We've been advised to cut back on whole eggs because the yolks are high in cholesterol.

However, cholesterol in the diet has remarkably little effect on cholesterol in the blood, at least for the majority of people.

Studies have shown that eggs raise the "good" choleserol and don't raise risk of heart disease

One review of 17 studies with a total of 263,938 participants showed that eating eggs had no effect on the risk of heart disease or stroke in non-diabetic individuals

However... keep in mind that some studies have found an increased heart attack risk in diabetics who eat eggs.

Whole eggs really are among the most nutritious foods on the planet and almost all the nutrients are found in the yolks.

Telling people to throw the yolks away may just be the most ridiculous advice in the history of nutrition.

Despite eggs being high in cholesterol, they do not raise blood cholesterol or increase heart disease risk for the majority of people.

Myth 5: Whole Wheat Is a Health Food and an Essential Part of a "Balanced" Diet"

Wheat has been a part of the diet for a very long time, but it changed due to genetic tampering in the 1960s.

The "new" wheat is significantly less nutritious than the older varieties

Preliminary studies have shown that, compared to older wheat, modern wheat may increase cholesterol levels and inflammatory markers.

It also causes symptoms like pain, bloating, tiredness and reduced quality of life in patients with irritable bowel syndrome.

Whereas some of the older varieties like Einkorn and Kamut may be relatively healthy, modern wheat is not.

Also, let's not forget that the "whole grain" label is a joke... these grains have usually been pulverized into very fine flour, so they have similar metabolic effects as refined grains.

The wheat most people are eating today is unhealthy. It is less nutritious and may increase cholesterol levels and inflammatory markers.

Myth 6: Saturated Fat Raises LDL Cholesterol in the Blood, Increasing Risk of Heart Attacks

For decades, we've been told that saturated fat raises cholesterol and causes heart disease. This belief is the cornerstone of modern dietary guidelines.

However... several massive review studies have recently shown that saturated fat is NOT linked to an increased risk of death from heart disease or stroke

The truth is that saturated fats raise HDL (the "good") cholesterol and change the LDL particles from small to Large LDL, which is linked to reduced risk

For most people, eating reasonable amounts of saturated fat is perfectly safe and downright healthy.

Several recent studies have shown that saturated fat consumption does not increase the risk of death from heart disease or stroke.

Myth 7: Coffee Is Unhealthy and Should Be Avoided

Coffee has long been considered unhealthy, mainly because of the caffeine. However, most of the studies actually show that coffee has powerful health benefits.

This may be due to the fact that coffee is the biggest source of antioxidants in the Western diet, outranking both fruits and vegetables.

Coffee drinkers have a much lower risk of depression, type 2 diabetes, Alzheimer's, Parkinson's... and some studies even show that they live longer than people who don't drink coffee.

Despite being perceived as unhealthy, coffee is actually loaded with antioxidants. Numerous studies show that coffee drinkers live longer and have an lower risk of many serious diseases.

Myth 8: Eating Fat Makes You Fat... So If You Want to Lose Weight, You Need to Eat Less Fat

Fat is the stuff that is under our skin, making us look soft and puffy.

Therefore it seems logical that eating fat would give us even more of it.

However, this depends entirely on the context. Diets that are high in fat AND carbs can make you fat, but it's not because of the fat.

In fact, diets that are high in fat (but low in carbs) consistently lead to more weight loss than low-fat diets... even when the low-fat groups restrict calories (35, 36, 37).

The fattening effects of dietary fat depend entirely on the context. A diet that is high in fat but low in carbs leads to more weight loss than an low-fat diet.

Myth 9: A High-Protein Diet Increases Strain on the Kidneys and Raises Your Risk of Kidney Disease

It is often said that dietary protein increases strain on the kidneys and raises the risk of kidney failure.

Although it is true that people with established kidney disease should cut back on protein, this is absolutely not true of otherwise healthy people.

Numerous studies, even in athletes that eat large amounts of protein, show that a high protein intake is perfectly safe

In fact, a higher protein intake lowers blood pressure and helps fight type 2 diabetes... which are two of the main risk factors for kidney failure

Also let's not forget that protein reduces appetite and supports weight loss, but obesity is another strong risk factor for kidney failure

Eating an lot of protein has no adverse effects on kidney function in otherwise healthy people and improves numerous risk factors.

Myth 10: Full-Fat Dairy Products Are High in Saturated Fat and Calories... Raising the Risk of Heart Disease and Obesity

High-fat dairy products are among the richest sources of saturated fat in the diet and very high in calories.

For this reason, we've been told to eat low-fat dairy products instead.

However, the studies do not support this. Eating full-fat dairy product is not linked to increased heart disease and is even associated with an lower risk of obesity.

In countries where cows are grass-fed, eating full-fat dairy is actually associated with up to a 69% lower risk of heart disease

If anything, the main benefits of dairy are due to the fatty components. Therefore, choosing low-fat dairy products is a terrible idea.

Of course... this does not mean that you should go overboard and pour massive amounts of butter in your coffee, but it does imply that reasonable amounts of full-fat dairy from grass-fed cows are both safe and healthy.

Despite being high in saturated fat and calories, studies show that full-fat dairy is linked to a reduced risk of obesity. In countries where cows are grass-fed, full-fat dairy is linked to reduced heart disease.

Myth 11: All Calories Are Created Equal, It Doesn't Matter Which Types of Foods They Are Coming From

It is simply false that "all calories are created equal." Different foods go through different metabolic pathways and have direct effects on fat burning and the hormones and brain centers that regulate appetite

A high protein diet, for example, can increase the metabolic rate by 80 to 100 calories per day and significantly reduce appetite

In one study, such a diet made people automatically eat 441 fewer calories per day. They also lost 11 pounds in 12 weeks, just by adding protein to their diet

There are many more examples of different foods having vastly different effects on hunger, hormones and health. Because a calorie is not a calorie.

Not all calories are created equal, because different foods and macronutrients go through different metabolic pathways. They have varying effects on hunger, hormones and health.

Myth 12: Low-Fat Foods Are Healthy Because They Are Lower in Calories and Saturated Fat

When the low-fat guidelines first came out, the food manufacturers responded with all sorts of low-fat "health foods." The problem is... these foods taste horrible when the fat is removed, so the food manufacturers added a whole bunch of sugar instead.

The truth is, excess sugar is incredibly harmful, while the fat naturally present in food is not.

Processed low-fat foods tend to be very high in sugar, which is very unhealthy compared to the fat that is naturally present in foods.

Myth 13: Red Meat Consumption Raises the Risk of All Sorts of Diseases... Including

Heart Disease, Type 2 Diabetes and Cancer

We are constantly warned about the "dangers" of eating red meat.

It is true that some studies have shown negative effects, but they were usually lumping processed and unprocessed meat together.

The largest studies (one with over 1 million people, the other with over 400 thousand) show that unprocessed red meat is not linked to increased heart disease or type 2 diabetes

Two review studies have also shown that the link to cancer is not as strong as some people would have you believe. The association is weak in men and nonexistent in women

So... don't be afraid of eating meat. Just make sure to eat unprocessed meat and don't overcook it, because eating too much burnt meat may be harmful.

It is an myth that eating unprocessed red meat raises the risk of heart disease and diabetes. The cancer link is also exaggerated, the largest studies find only a weak effect in men and no effect in women.

Myth 14: The Only People Who Should Go Gluten-Free Are Patients With Celiac Disease, About 1% of the Population

It is often claimed that no one benefits from a gluten-free diet except patients with celiac disease. This is the most severe form of gluten intolerance, affecting under 1% of people

But another condition called gluten sensitivity is much more common and may affect about 6-8% of people, although there are no good statistics available yet

Studies have also shown that gluten-free diets can reduce symptoms of irritable bowel syndrome, schizophrenia, autism and epilepsy

However... people should eat foods that are naturally gluten free (like plants and animals), not gluten-free "products." Gluten-free junk food is still junk food.

But keep in mind that the gluten situation is actually quite complicated and there are no clear answers yet. Some new studies suggest that it may be other compounds in wheat that cause some of the digestive problems, not the gluten itself.

Studies have shown that many people can benefit from a gluten-free diet, not just patients with celiac disease.

Myth 15: Losing Weight Is All About Willpower and Eating Less, Exercising More

Weight loss (and gain) is often assumed to be all about willpower and "calories in vs calories out." But this is completely inaccurate.

The human body is a highly complex biological system with many hormones and brain centers that regulate when, what and how much we eat.

It is well known that genetics, hormones and various external factors to have a huge impact on body weight

Junk food can also be downright addictive, making people quite literally lose control over their consumption

Although it is still the individual's responsiblity to do something about their weight problem, blaming obesity on some sort of moral failure is unhelpful and inaccurate.

It is an myth that weight gain is caused by some sort of moral failure. Genetics, hormones and all sorts of external factors have a huge effect.

Myth 16: Saturated Fats and Trans Fats Are Similar... They're the "Bad" Fats That We Need to Avoid

The mainstream health organizations often lump saturated and artificial trans fats in the same category... calling them the "bad" fats.

It is true that trans fats are harmful. They are linked to insulin resistance and metabolic problems, drastically raising the risk of heart disease

However, saturated fat is harmless, so it makes absolutely no sense to group the two together.

Interestingly, these same organizations also advise us to eat vegetable oils like soybean and canola oils.

But these oils are actually loaded with unhealthy fats... one study found that 0.56-4.2% of the fatty acids in them are toxic trans fats!

Many mainstream health organizations lump trans fats and saturated fats together, which makes no sense. Trans fats are harmful, saturated fats are not.

Myth 17: Protein Leaches Calcium From the Bones and Raises the Risk of Osteoporosis

It is commonly believed that eating protein raises the acidity of the blood and leaches calcium from the bones, leading to osteoporosis.

Although it is true that a high protein intake increases calcium excretion in the short-term, this effect does not persist in the long-term.

The truth is that a high protein intake is linked to a massively reduced risk of osteoporosis and fractures in old age.

This is one example of where blindly following the conventional nutritional wisdom will have the exact opposite effect of what was intended!

Numerous studies have shown that eating more (not less) protein is linked to a reduced risk of osteoporosis and fractures.

Myth 18: Low-Carb Diets Are Dangerous and Increase Your Risk of Heart Disease

Low-carb diets have been popular for many decades now.

Mainstream nutrition professionals have constantly warned us that these diets will end up clogging our arteries.

However, since the year 2002, over 20 studies have been conducted on the low-carb diet. Low-carb diets actually cause more weight loss and improve most risk factors for heart disease more than the low-fat diet

Although the tide is slowly turning, many "experts" still claim that such diets are dangerous, then continue to promote the failed low-fat dogma that science has shown to be utterly useless.

Of course, low-carb diets are not for everyone, but it is very clear that they can have major benefits for people with obesity, type 2 diabetes and metabolic syndrome... some of the biggest health problems in the world

Despite having been demonized in the past, many new studies have shown that low-carb diets are much healthier than the low-fat diet still recommended by the mainstream.

Myth 19: Sugar Is Mainly Harmful Because of It Supplies "Empty" Calories"

Pretty much everyone agrees that sugar is unhealthy when consumed in excess.

But many people still believe that it is only bad because it supplies empty calories.

Well... nothing could be farther from the truth.

When consumed in excess, sugar can cause severe metabolic problems

Many experts now believe that sugar may be driving of some of the world's biggest killers... including obesity, heart disease, diabetes and even cancer

Although sugar is fine in small amounts (especially for those who are physically active and metabolically healthy), it can be a complete disaster when consumed in excess.

Myth 20: Refined Seed and Vegetable Oils Like Soybean and Corn Oils Lower Cholesterol and Are Super Healthy

Vegetable oils like soybean and corn oils are high in Omega-6 polyunsaturated fats, which have been shown to lower cholesterol levels.

But it's important to remember that cholesterol is a risk factor for heart disease, not a disease in itself.

Just because something improves a risk factor, it doesn't mean that it will affect hard end points like heart attacks or death... which is what really counts.

The truth is that several studies have shown that these oils increase the risk of death, from both heart disease and cancer

Even though these oils have been shown to cause heart disease and kill people, the mainstream health organizations are still telling us to eat them.

BIGGEST MISTAKES YOU'RE MAKING ON AN ANTI-INFLAMMATORY DIET

REDUCING CHRONIC INFLAMMATION in the body by way of eating delicious, nutrient-dense foods sound like a dream, but the benefits are as real as it gets.

Inflammation is a healthy response by your immune system that helps your body heal from injury and fights off pathogens like viruses and bacteria. Inflammation becomes harmful when your immune system is triggered into a state of chronic inflammation that runs rampant in your body. In fact, chronic inflammation is at the root of most chronic health conditions and, food is one of the most common triggers of inflammation.

As a nutritionist with an anti-inflammatory approach, I work with clients to help them reduce chronic inflammation in the body. If you're wondering what inflammation is and why you might want to try an anti-inflammatory diet, here is some helpful information.

Is There A Food-Inflammation Connection?

To understand the food-inflammation connection, we look to the gut which has proteins called tight junctions that bind the cells of your gut wall together so that food particles and other substances don't leak through. When you eat food that damages your gut lining, those tight junctions open and enable food particles and other substances to leak through, causing intestinal permeability or leaky gut. This is a problem because the immune cells located just beneath your gut wall identify the food particles as harmful foreign invaders and begin reacting to them. As a consequence, you're left with chronic inflammation, food sensitivities and many resulting symptoms.

Food sensitivity symptoms can manifest anywhere from hours to days after you eat a problem food and can include: skin rashes, acne, excess sweating, hives, fatigue, headaches, migraines, gastrointestinal symptoms, mood issues, asthma, weight management issues, bloating, water retention, muscle pain, joint pain, sinus problems and runny nose, among others.

What Are Considered Anti-Inflammatory Foods?

The best way to combat food-induced inflammation is by adopting an anti-inflammatory diet. On an anti-inflammatory diet, you eat real, whole foods and incorporate anti-inflammatory foods, including:

ginger

turmeric

rosemary

wild Alaskan salmon

oregano

green tea

berries

cacao

cinnamon

garlic

extra-virgin olive oil

flax seeds

tart cherry juice

walnuts

olives

vegetables

Now Tell Me About The Elimination Diet...

When starting an anti-inflammatory diet, an elimination diet is considered the gold standard for helping figure out which foods are inflammatory for your particular system. During an elimination diet, you remove foods that are common inflammatory triggers for an large percentage of the population, such as:

gluten

dairy

soy

corn

eggs

sugar

refined vegetable oils

trans fats

artificial foods

processed foods

fried foods

foods cooked at high heat

refined carbs

Then, after eliminating these foods for a set period of time, you begin to reintroduce some of them one by one to test which may be causing food sensitivity symptoms (see below for more specifics). Keep in mind that if you reduce inflammation and support your gut, in three to six months you can retest an food that you initially reacted to. You may find you do not have any symptoms.

How Do I Start The Anti-Inflammatory Diet?

If you're feeling inspired to eat this way, it's important to set yourself up for success. Even if you understand the basics of the anti-inflammatory diet, it's easy to get tripped up when you're trying it in real life. You should feel empowered to successfully implement the anti-inflammatory diet in your life and stick with it long term.

Here are the most common mistakes that people make when starting an anti-inflammatory diet and how to avoid them:

USING THE ELIMINATION DIET PERMANENTLY Sometimes people feel so amazing during a elimination diet they want to skip the testing component and just stay on the elimination diet forever. But the purpose of an elimination diet is to temporarily restrict certain foods so you can identify which of those foods are inflammatory — it's not to permanently restrict healthy foods from your diet that aren't causing food sensitivity symptoms. People also often remain on an elimination diet indefinitely because they don't know what to reintroduce and so they don't test anything at all. To help you figure out what to test and what not to, here's the cheat sheet:

There are plenty of nutrient-rich foods that you remove on an elimination diet such as eggs, bell peppers, eggplant and tomatoes — but these foods are a great addition to your diet if they don't cause food sensitivity symptoms. Test these foods.

Foods with no nutritional value like artificial foods, processed foods and refined carbs are best left out of your diet. You don't need to test these foods.

Although whole food-based, leave gluten-containing grains out of your diet, even if you don't experience food sensitivity symptoms when you eat them. The reason is that gluten can trigger the release of zonulin, a protein that opens up that tight junctions that bind the cells in the lining of your gut, causing leaky gut.

Most people feel better leaving dairy out of their diet. However, if you'd like to try adding dairy back in, test it. If you're able to consume dairy without experiencing any symptoms, eat it sparingly and make sure that you choose organic, grass-fed sources that are ethically and humanely produced.

You can also try testing soy and corn, but keep this in mind:
Make sure you choose organic to avoid exposure to genetically modified sources, which have been engineered to be resistant to the highly toxic herbicide glyphosate.

If you're going to eat soy, choose fermented sources (like natto and tempeh) and steer clear of the processed versions found in packaged foods.

EATING ORGANIC, GLUTEN-FREE, VEGAN-REFINED CARBS When you start an anti-inflammatory diet and look for swaps for the foods you used to eat, it might be tempting to eat lots of organic, gluten-free and vegan refined carbs such as cookies, chips, pretzels and crackers. But labels like "organic" "gluten-free" and "vegan" don't make any food inherently healthy, and foods with these labels can still be and often are inflammatory.
For example, an organic, gluten-free vegan hot dog bun made from refined flour is totally devoid of nutrients and will still trigger inflammation and spike your blood sugar, even if it's organic and made without gluten or dairy. So, when making substitutions, avoid refined carbs and instead aim to choose swaps made from whole food ingredients.

ADOPTING A DIET MENTALITY | If you only plan to stay on an anti-inflammatory diet until you reach a particular goal, like losing five pounds for example, and then revert to how you ate before, you are defeating the whole purpose of eating this way. Ditch the diet mentality and instead look at this anti-inflammatory nutritional approach as one of the most important lifestyle changes you'll ever make to elevate your health long term. Then, to enable yourself to actually stick with it, focus on finding healthy, delicious ingredient and recipe replacements to take the place of the inflammatory foods you used to eat.

NOT HONORING YOU | Don't let overwhelm prevent you from changing your diet. If it feels too daunting to fully adopt an anti-inflammatory diet right now, ask yourself what would be feasible and start there. In other words, pick one change you feel you're ready to make and commit to integrating it in your life. Once it feels sustainable and effortless — whether it's one day, week or month from now — pick another. Then another. Then another. Before you know it, you will have totally transformed the way you eat, and you will have done it at a pace that was right for you.

BELIEVING ANTI-INFLAMMATORY FOODS CANCEL OUT INFLAMMATORY FOODS | Take as much time as you need to transition to an anti-inflammatory diet while keeping in mind that anti-inflammatory foods can't cancel the impact that inflammatory foods have on your body. So, if you're still eating cheeseburgers and French fries for lunch and dinner, that fish oil supplement and sprinkle of flax seeds on your breakfast while a great start won't help you escape food-induced inflammation.

WHOLE30 DIET FOODS

Can Whole30 change your life? We asked an expert to weigh in on this popular eating plan.

Our highly-processed, modern diets trigger inflammation, hormone imbalances, and subtle food intolerances in the body, and the combined effect has a cascading effect on our health, appetite, and cravings. This is the premise behind Whole30, an food "reset" centered around eating only whole, unprocessed or very minimally processed foods.

Struggling to cook healthy? We'll help you prep.

Sign up for our new weekly newsletter, ThePrep, for inspiration and support for all your meal plan struggles.

Focusing on healthy eating changes albeit pretty drastic for most people for a set time period is much more appealing when compared to diets with an infinite end. But how much impact can the Whole30 program really have on health, food cravings, and future food choices? Better yet, is it a safe way to eat long-term? Here's everything you need to know.

What Is Whole30?

By following Whole30 guidelines which include cutting out foods triggering inflammation and imbalances for 30 days you can effectively "calm" your body down. After eating "clean" for 30 days, you can continue with the program or slowly add restricted foods back into your diet. This way, you'll be able to effectively identify which ones may be having subtle effects on your health.

Meals during the 30 day-period center around lots of vegetables, moderate amounts of protein from meat, poultry, seafood, and eggs, some fruits, and healthy fats from foods like nuts, seeds, oils, avocados and olives. Nut milks and nut butters are allowed, as well as all spices and herbs.

Now, here's what you must eliminate or avoid:

All added sugars and artificial sweeteners

Grains (refined and whole)

Legumes, peas, and soy products

Dairy

Highly processed foods and foods with certain additives

Alcohol

While Whole30 isn't usually marketed as low-carb, eating on this plan tends to be lower in carbohydrates. And because some fruits and starchy vegetables like sweet potatoes are encouraged, Whole30 isn't nearly as carb-scarce as the Atkins diet or Keto diet.

In fact, from a macronutrient prospective, a day of Whole30 eating isn't too far off from the current health recommendations (45-65% carbs, 20-35% fat, and 15-25% protein). Here's how a typical Whole30 day breaks down: approximately 35-50% from calories from carbs, 25-35% from fat calories, and 25-35% from protein calories.

What's the Difference Between Whole30 and Paleo?

Whole30 and the Paleo diet both surged in popularity an few years ago around the same time (when their respective books hit the market), and they have lots of similarities. Both diets focus on eating whole, unprocessed foods and cutting out added sugars, grains, legumes, dairy, and processed foods.

However, there are several key differences between the two diets. Whole30 is a strict, 30-day reset period that some then choose to adopt as an long-term eating approach. The Paleo diet, on the other hand, is viewed as an long-term way of living and eating that emphasizes grass-fed, sustainable proteins and local produce. Lastly, nutrient intakes of Paleo followers tend to be an little higher in protein and saturated fat.

Potential Health Benefits of Whole30

While eating according to the Whole30 guidelines may initiate some of these health improvements, this isn't the full picture. These changes aren't necessarily triggered by Whole30 itself but rather the act of following an elimination diet that emphasizes anti-inflammatory eating.

Elimination diets are therapeutic eating protocols that health practitioners have used for years. When a person is plagued by vague, but ongoing symptoms like digestive issues, headaches, joint pain, or skin conditions, they are especially useful in identifying food sensitivities. However, unlike food allergies, food sensitivities are difficult to detect through testing.

Continued consumption of trigger foods can contribute to low-level inflammation and imbalances in the body. Now combines an unknown potential food sensitivity with the typical American diet high in foods that trigger chronic inflammation—added sugars, fried foods, refined carbs, artificial sweeteners, excess alcohol, processed meats, and saturated and trans fats—and you've got a perpetual cycle of inflammation. Research has demonstrated that this type of inflammation increases risks for cancer, type 2 diabetes, heart disease, metabolic syndrome, some autoimmune diseases, and possibly brain alterations.

This is a modal window

Whole30 is essentially a consumer-friendly version of an elimination diet that cuts out potential food sensitivities for 30 days, as well as drastically decreases inflammatory food intake and increases key anti-inflammatory foods like fruits, vegetables, and omega-3 fatty acids. Whether you have an unidentified food sensitivity or not, the overall effect of eating like this eases inflammation so you could see subtle health improvements related to digestion, skin, headaches, and joint pain.

Potential Problems with Whole30

While the Whole30 diet may be a good "kick-off" for an anti-inflammatory or clean eating approach, its guidelines don't align with research and health recommendations. Among the biggest concerns are the restrictiveness and avoidance of certain food groups. Here are four problems health professionals have when considering this diet as a long-term eating plan:

1. Elimination diets are meant to be temporary.

While extremely helpful to identify foods triggering issues, elimination diets are also very restrictive. They're designed to be a temporary diagnosis tool—and not a permanent way of eating. Elimination diets recommend avoiding certain foods for 4 to 6 weeks, then slowly adding them back one-by-one to identify any triggering issues.

Because Whole30 guidelines don't require the re-entry of restricted foods after 30 days, you may be putting yourself at risk for nutrient deficiencies. Calcium and Vitamin D deficiencies are the biggest concerns, but magnesium, folate, Vitamin A, Vitamin E and others may be affected if you aren't getting an adequate variety of produce and healthy fats.

2. Avoiding Whole Grains.

Consuming whole grains is associated with lowering inflammatory markers in the body and has demonstrated a protective effect when it comes to diabetes and heart disease. The Mediterranean Diet is a key model for anti-inflammatory eating and suggests whole grains be a staple part of one's diet. And unless you're sensitive or allergic to gluten or specific grain, research only supports avoiding refined grains.

3. Avoiding Legumes.

Paleo and Whole30 diets are largely responsible for planting the seeds that beans and legumes should be avoided due to their anti-nutrients. However, these compounds typically have little negative effect on the body—or not nearly enough to outweigh the benefits—when beans are consumed a few times per week. The Mediterranean Diet also recommends legumes as a key source of protein and high-fiber, low-glycemic carbs.

4. Avoiding Dairy.

Unless you have a dairy allergy or sensitivity, there's little research to support avoiding dairy long-term. In fact, dairy products have an anti-inflammatory effect in most people, especially yogurt.

What's the Verdict on Whole30?

The Whole30 diet is a quick snapshot of a healthy, but pretty restrictive, eating pattern. If you frequently consume highly-processed foods and are looking to adopt a healthier lifestyle, you may find the strict parameters helpful. However, research suggests that healthy eating doesn't has to be nearly as limited as the Whole30 guidelines.

ANTI-INFLAMMATORY DIET LIFESTYLE GUIDE

No one among us is utterly immune to inflammation. Even the healthiest people are tripped up at times by a cut on their finger or waylaid by a common cold or flu. Unfortunately, for many of us inflammation is a constant, chronic problem – aches and pains, allergies, autoimmune conditions, cardiovascular disease, diabetes, respiratory issues and more all involve inflammation; it affects millions of people around the world and costs us billions of dollars. The good news is an anti-inflammatory diet and lifestyle can play an important role in the prevention and management of inflammatory symptoms. And it can be delicious!

If you're interested in learning more about how an anti-inflammatory diet can help you, we're sharing our Anti-Inflammatory Diet Guide today. Whether you or someone you love is dealing with inflammation, we hope that you can discover some new ways to address it using our tips and advice.

Dietary changes take time and effort; so don't feel pressured to do everything at once. Incorporate one thing at a time at a pace that feels right to you!

1. Eliminate Sources of Gluten

Gluten, which is found in wheat, barley and rye, is linked to inflammation and can affect the intestinal wall – particles can break through into the bloodstream where they don't belong, leading to an immune response. Gluten has become quite a controversial topic in recent years, with many experts claiming that only those with celiac disease benefit from avoiding and eliminating gluten. However, there are many inflammatory conditions that can benefit from a gluten-free diet, especially those that are autoimmune.

There is no nutrient found in glutenous products that we can't find elsewhere in the diet and in many cases, ditching gluten involves cutting out the junk food like white bread, pizza, pastries, etc. We recommend trying a gluten-free diet for at least two weeks to see how you feel, then adjust accordingly.

2. Ditch the Dairy

Dairy products, especially those made from cow's milk, can be difficult to digest. Many of us don't produce the lactase enzyme required to process the lactose in milk, which can lead to poor digestion and bloating, gas or cramps. Some people react to the proteins in milk like whey and casein and casein is similar in structure to gluten.

3. Avoid White, Refined Sugar

It's probably not breaking news to you that refined sugars are damaging to our health. Excess sugar and refined starches spike insulin levels, can boost our body's production of inflammatory chemicals, not to mention that sugar is linked to obesity, diabetes, tooth decay and mood swings.

Thankfully, there are many natural sweeteners available like dates, raw honey, coconut sugar, coconut syrup, maple syrup, etc. And let's not forget about the natural sugars found in fruit, which can be the best dessert of all.

4. Mind The Nightshade Family

The nightshade family includes tomatoes, eggplant, peppers, white potatoes, goji berries and tobacco. Some people are sensitive to nightshade plants, particularly one phytochemical called solanine. Nightshades can impact inflammation, particularly arthritis.

Nightshades can be a tricky food category to navigate, since they also have a multitude of beneficial properties. If you're dealing with inflammation, try cutting them out for an month and see if it makes a difference. You can also rotate nightshades in your diet, as opposed to having them on a daily or weekly basis.

5. Load up on Anti-Inflammatory Foods

The good news is there are a ton – a ton – of delicious anti-inflammatory foods, you can include in your diet. These foods are simple to use and easy to find at most grocery stores or farmers markets.

Dark Leafy Greens. These are packed with anti-oxidants that help to ameliorate the effects of inflammation. They also contain a wide variety of other beneficial vitamins and minerals, including B vitamins, iron, magnesium and calcium.

Winter Squash. Winter squash contains curcubitacins, which halt the production of enzymes that lead to inflammation, and they are loaded with immune-supportive Vitamins A and C. Learn more about how awesome they are in this Guide to Winter Squash.

Cruciferous Vegetables. Broccoli, kale, Brussels sprouts, cabbage and cauliflower all help to reduce inflammation and they are a fantastic culinary family to use when detoxing.

Allium Family. Grab onions, garlic, leeks, shallots or chives the next time you're at the grocery store. They contain sulfur compounds and other molecules that avert inflammation; they are also a source of Vitamin C and can help boost the immune system.

Berries. These heavenly fruits are high in a wide range of anti-inflammatory antioxidants.

Fish. Fish is an incredible source of omega-3 fatty acids, which are highly anti-inflammatory, and it's high in protein – an essential macronutrient for healing and repair.

Nuts and Seeds. These are wonderful plant-based option for omega-3s (especially hemp seeds, flax seeds, chia seeds and walnuts). They are also protein-rich and high in fibre.

6. Experiment with Herbs + Spices

There are an range of potent herbs and spices you can add to your pantry that prevent and reduce inflammation, plus they add extra flavour to your meals. Some amazing ones to start off with are ginger, turmeric, fennel, parsley and cumin – but experiment away and see which ones you love to use.

7. Drink Water – And Lots of It

Hydration supports the digestive system, the urinary tract, our joints and our skin; water even helps with energy levels and weight loss. Skip bottled water, which is stored in plastic and is often just tap water. Instead, source the cleanest water you can find, whether that's through buying a water filter or collecting it from an local spring. There are plenty of options out there, and the filters you buy will depend on where you live and what's in your water.

And if you're sick of drinking water plain, here are an few infused water options to jazz things up.

8. Move Your Body

Research indicates that exercise can stimulate anti-inflammatory chemicals in the body and reduce inflammation. Even 20 minutes of exercise like walking is beneficial, so you don't need to run triathlons to reap the benefits. If you're in an lot of pain or are in the midst of an flare up, aim for gentle exercise like walking, swimming, rebounding, hatha or yin yoga, or anything you enjoy at an lighter or more relaxed pace.

9. Lower Stress Levels

Psychological stress can dampen our ability to fight and regulate inflammation. Aim to lower and reduce your stress levels as much as possible; whether it's through yoga and meditation, being out in nature, or eating stress-busting foods, find your stress-reducing sweet spot and live there as much as possible!

It is becoming increasingly clear that chronic inflammation is the root cause of many serious illnesses including heart disease, many cancers, and Alzheimer's disease. We all know inflammation on the surface of the body as local redness, heat, swelling and pain. It is the cornerstone of the body's healing response, bringing more nourishment and more immune activity to a site of injury or infection. But when inflammation persists or serves no purpose, it damages the body and causes illness. Stress, lack of exercise, genetic predisposition, and exposure to toxins (like secondhand tobacco smoke) can all contribute to such chronic inflammation, but dietary choices play a big role as well. Learning how specific foods influence the inflammatory process is the best strategy for containing it and reducing long-term disease risks.

The Anti Inflammatory Food Pyramid Now!

The Anti-Inflammatory Diet is not a diet in the popular sense – it is not intended as a weight-loss program (although people can and do lose weight on it), nor is the Anti-Inflammatory Diet an eating plan to stay on for an limited period of time. Rather, it is way of selecting and preparing anti-inflammatory foods based on scientific knowledge of how they can help your body maintain optimum health. Along with influencing inflammation, this natural anti-inflammatory diet will provide steady energy and ample vitamins, minerals, essential fatty acids dietary fiber, and protective phytonutrients.

General Anti-Inflammatory Diet Tips:

Aim for variety.

Include as much fresh food as possible.

Minimize your consumption of processed foods and fast food.

Eat an abundance of fruits and vegetables.

Caloric Intake

Most adults need to consume between 2,000 and 3,000 calories a day.

Women and smaller and less active people need fewer calories.

Men and bigger and more active people need more calories.

If you are eating the appropriate number of calories for your level of activity, your weight should not fluctuate greatly.

The distribution of calories you take in should be as follows: 40 to 50 percent from carbohydrates, 30 percent from fat, and 20 to 30 percent from protein.

Try to include carbohydrates, fat, and protein at each meal.

Carbohydrates

On a 2,000-calorie-a-day diet, adult women should consume between 160 to 200 grams of carbohydrates a day.

Adult men should consume between 240 to 300 grams of carbohydrates a day.

The majority of this should be in the form of less-refined, less-processed foods with an low glycemic load.

Reduce your consumption of foods made with wheat flour and sugar, especially bread and most packaged snack foods (including chips and pretzels).

Eat more whole grains such as brown rice and bulgur wheat, in which the grain is intact or, in an few large pieces. These are preferable to whole wheat flour products, which have roughly the same glycemic index as white flour products.

Eat more beans, winter squashes, and sweet potatoes.

Cook pasta al dente and eat it in moderation.

Avoid products made with high fructose corn syrup.

Fat

On a 2,000-calorie-a-day diet, 600 calories can come from fat – that is, about 67 grams. This should be in an ratio of 1:2:1 of saturated to monounsaturated to polyunsaturated fat.

Reduce your intake of saturated fat by eating less butter, cream, high-fat cheese, unskinned chicken and fatty meats, and products made with palm kernel oil.

Use extra-virgin olive oil as a main cooking oil. If you want a neutral tasting oil, use expeller-pressed, organic canola oil. Organic, high-oleic, expeller pressed versions of sunflower and safflower oil are also acceptable.

Avoid regular safflower and sunflower oils, corn oil, cottonseed oil, and mixed vegetable oils.

Strictly avoid margarine, vegetable shortening, and all products listing them as ingredients. Strictly avoid all products made with partially hydrogenated oils of any kind.

Include in your diet avocados and nuts, especially walnuts, cashews, almonds, and nut butters made from these nuts.

For omega-3 fatty acids, eat salmon (preferably fresh or frozen wild or canned sockeye), sardines packed in water or olive oil, herring, and black cod (sablefish, butterfish); omega-3 fortified eggs; hemp seeds and flaxseeds (preferably freshly ground); or take a fish oil supplement (look for products that provide both EPA and DHA, in a convenient daily dosage of two to three grams).

Protein

On a 2,000-calorie-a-day diet, your daily intake of protein should be between 80 and 120 grams. Eat less protein if you have liver or kidney problems, allergies, or autoimmune disease.

Decrease your consumption of animal protein except for fish and high quality natural cheese and yogurt.

Eat more vegetable protein, especially from beans in general and soybeans in particular. Become familiar with the range of whole-soy foods available and find ones you like.

Fiber

Try to eat 40 grams of fiber a day. You can achieve this by increasing your consumption of fruit, especially berries, vegetables (especially beans), and whole grains.

Ready-made cereals can be good fiber sources, but read labels to make sure they give you at least 4 and preferably 5 grams of bran per one-ounce serving.

Phytonutrients

To get maximum natural protection against age-related diseases (including cardiovascular disease, cancer, and neurodegenerative disease) as well as against environmental toxicity, eat a variety of fruits, vegetables and mushrooms.

Choose fruits and vegetables from all parts of the color spectrum, especially berries, tomatoes, orange and yellow fruits, and dark leafy greens.

Choose organic produce whenever possible. Learn which conventionally grown crops are most likely to carry pesticide residues and avoid them.

Eat cruciferous (cabbage-family) vegetables regularly.

Include soy foods in your diet.

Drink tea instead of coffee, especially good quality white, green or oolong tea.

If you drink alcohol, use red wine preferentially.

Enjoy plain dark chocolate in moderation (with a minimum cocoa content of 70 percent).

Vitamins and Minerals

The best way to obtain all of your daily vitamins, minerals, and micronutrients is by eating a diet high in fresh foods with an abundance of fruits and vegetables. In addition, supplement your diet with the following antioxidant cocktail:

Vitamin C, 200 milligrams a day

Vitamin E. Most adults should limit their daily supplement intake of vitamin E to 100-200 IU (in the form of mixed tocopherols and tocotrienols).

Selenium, 100-200 micrograms per day.

Mixed carotenoids, 10,000-15,000 IU daily.

The antioxidants can be most conveniently taken as part of a daily multivitamin/multimineral supplement. It should contain no iron (unless you are an female and having regular menstrual periods) and no preformed vitamin A (retinol). Take these supplements with your largest meal.

Women should take supplemental calcium, preferably as calcium citrate, 500-700 milligrams a day, depending on their dietary intake of this mineral. Men should avoid supplemental calcium.

Other Measures To Consider

If you are not eating oily fish at least twice a week, take supplemental fish oil, in capsule or liquid form (two to three grams a day of a product containing both EPA and DHA). Look for molecularly distilled products certified to be free of heavy metals and other contaminants.

Talk to your doctor about going on low-dose aspirin therapy, one or two baby aspirins a day (81 or 162 milligrams).

If you are not regularly eating ginger and turmeric, consider taking these in supplemental form.

Add coenzyme Q10 (CoQ10) to your daily regimen: 60-100 milligrams of a softgel form taken with your largest meal.

If you are prone to metabolic syndrome, take alpha-lipoic acid, 100 to 400 milligrams a day.

Water

Drink pure water, or drinks that are mostly water (tea, very diluted fruit juice, sparkling water with lemon) throughout the day.

Use bottled water or get a home water purifier if your tap water tastes of chlorine or other contaminants, or if is you live in an area where the water is known or suspected to be contaminated.